# 5 ½ WAYS

## — TO —

# WELL-BEING

*A Comprehensive Lifestyle Medicine Prescription
to Optimise Your Psychological Health, Prevent
Disease and Live with Vitality and Joy*

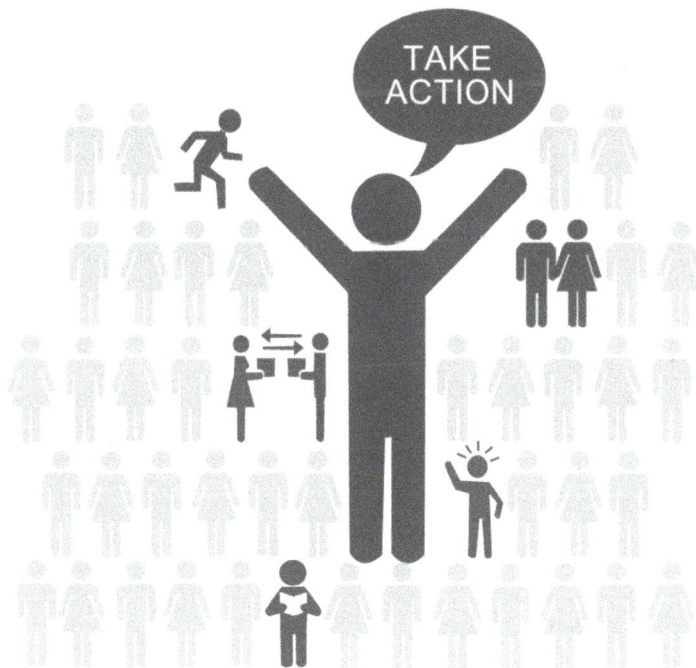

TAKE
ACTION

RUBEN S. SEETHARAMDOO PH.D.

The information, ideas, and suggestions in this book are not intended as a substitute for professional medical advice. Before following any suggestions contained in this book, you should consult your personal physician. Neither the author nor the publisher shall be liable or responsible for any loss or damage allegedly arising as a consequence of your use or application of any information or suggestions in this book.

Balboa Press books may be ordered through booksellers or by contacting:

Balboa Press
A Division of Hay House
1663 Liberty Drive
Bloomington, IN 47403
www.balboapress.com
1 (877) 407-4847

Because of the dynamic nature of the Internet, any web addresses or links contained in this book may have changed since publication and may no longer be valid. The views expressed in this work are solely those of the author and do not necessarily reflect the views of the publisher, and the publisher hereby disclaims any responsibility for them.

Any people depicted in stock imagery provided by Getty Images are models, and such images are being used for illustrative purposes only.
Certain stock imagery © Getty Images.

ISBN: 978-1-9822-8013-0 (sc)
ISBN: 978-1-9822-8014-7 (e)

Print information available on the last page.

Balboa Press rev. date: 08/14/2018

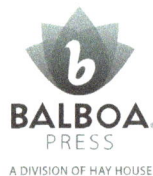

**BALBOA**
PRESS
A DIVISION OF HAY HOUSE

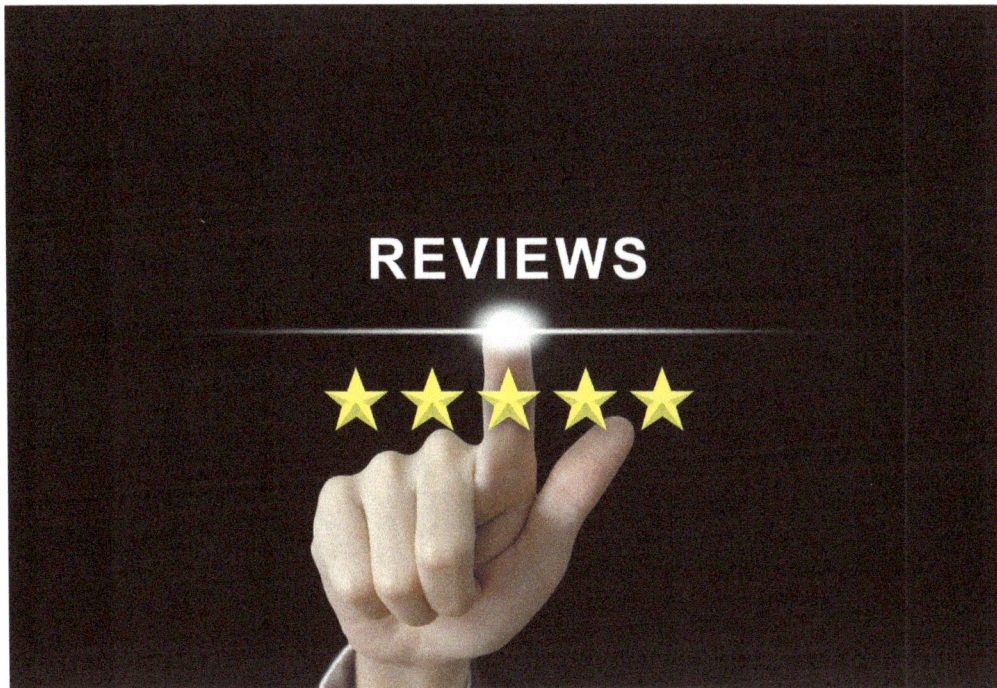

## REVIEWS

*What are health professionals saying about 5 1/2 ways to well-being?*

"I have spent 40+ years reading personal development/self-help books, and this is definitely one of the very best. Dr Seetharamdoo guides us through multifarious ways of dealing with how we sabotage ourselves from leading our best life. Illustrated with interesting examples and backed by the research of top professionals, as well as his own many years of practical experience helping people overcome self-imposed obstacles, he has created a resource that anybody can go back to again and again in their quest for wellbeing. The 1/2 of the 5 1/2 is what makes all the difference and his tips for how to stay motivated and engaged are invaluable."

**Sally Dyson**
**Addictions Directorate CNWL NHS Foundation Trust**
**Concertina Charitable Trust (Music for the Elderly) and Bodfach Trust**

"A great easy read book to help you increase your fulfilment in daily life. It provides a broad overview of the current thinking on happiness and wellbeing. It's as if you are having a personal coaching session."

**Dr Deepti Shah-Armon Clinical Director**

"I have really enjoyed reading the 5 ½ Ways to Well-being. It's a very useful resource for anyone wishing to improve their own health & well-being, as well as for those who are supporting others in making healthy lifestyle changes. The information is presented in a very accessible, positive way, providing plenty of inspiration and useful tips. It offers a path to wellness in manageable steps and inspires the confidence that anyone has it in them to achieve their 5 1/2 ways to well-being"

**Dina Potterton, Senior Occupational Therapist.**

"Educational, informative and well presented. In my opinion this book should be read by anyone who is interested in increasing their understanding of the science wellbeing, particularly those in the human development field.

**Mohammed Dualeh,Lead Group Facilitator, Recovery Day Programme**

"This is an exquisite and well written book on the important subject of wellbeing. It is concise, provides up to date information and is focused on how us as individuals can make positive changes to our wellbeing. The author combines his many years of experience to provide a holistic delivery of the contents. Open the book at a random page and you will find something useful to get you going. This book is for anybody with a keen interest in their own wellbeing or that of others. I highly recommend it."

**Azagun Marudamuthu, Senior Nurse Practitioner**

# Preface

Recently, I was humbled and honoured to receive the "Health Excellence Award" and also the "Health Coach of the Year" award in the UK by the Association of Professional Coaches, Trainers and Consultants. Since then, I have been approached by a lot of people asking me "what does a health coach do?" To answer this question, I have been using the metaphor below which I also use as my health and well-being manifesto.

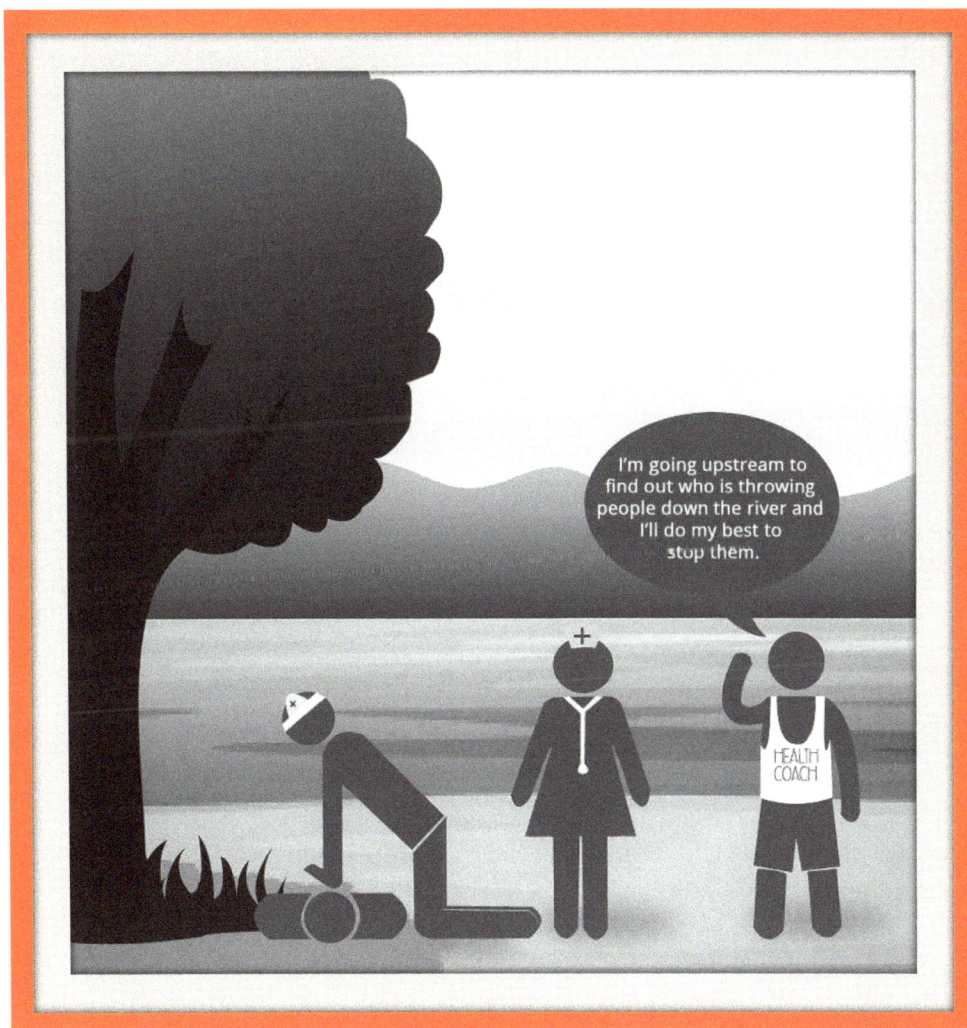

A doctor, nurse and a health coach were having a picnic by a riverbank, when a drowning lady floats into view, shouting for help. The doctor and the nurse leaps into the treacherous water and drags the lady out and perform cardio pulmonary resuscitation (CPR), thereby saving the lady's life. But before they can ask her what happened, a man floats by, also crying for help.

The doctor and nurse jump in the water again, drag him out to safety and resuscitate him. But as soon as he is safe and alive on the riverbank, two more people come floating down the river; children this time. The doctor and nurse are straight back in, rescuing them from the powerful current, but by now, they are starting to get tired. They turn to the health coach for help only to realise that he has turned his back. He's walking away from them, along the riverbank, towards the river's source.

All of a sudden the doctor and the nurse see four more people being swept down the river. "I need your help! Where are you going?" they shout to the health coach. The health coach turns to the doctor and the nurse and calmly replies, "I'm going upstream to find out who's throwing them in the river and get them to stop."

The doctor and nurse were dealing with the symptoms, while the health coach went looking for the cause. The fact is that most of common challenges that people in the health industry are struggling to overcome are actually symptoms. But when you try to solve the symptoms without dealing with the cause, it can be exhausting, frustrating, and ultimately fruitless.

The medical team—including doctors, nurses and support staff—do a brilliant and caring job to treat people's symptoms to make them better, but they are swamped and exhausted by the scale of the task and do not have time to deal with the root cause of these problems.

The UK government spends over £114 billion a year on the healthcare system, and most of that goes towards treating the symptoms of an illness (via drugs from pharmaceutical industries and surgery). Only 2-3 percent of the government's budget gets spent on treating the root cause of the problems, like addressing lifestyle (which is a genuine factor in overall health and well-being). Based on the current trend, if 97 percent of NHS budget is spent on treating illness, it should be rebranded as the "National Illness Service" and not the National Health Service. More investment needs to be allocated to lifestyle medicine. According to the American College of Lifestyle Medicine, "Lifestyle Medicine involves the use of evidence-based lifestyle therapeutic approaches, such as a predominantly whole food, plant-based diet, regular physical activity, adequate sleep, stress management, avoidance of risky substance use, and other non-drug modalities, to prevent, treat, and, oftentimes, reverse the lifestyle-related, chronic disease that's all too prevalent."

However, there is a light at the end of the tunnel, as the NHS has just celebrated its 70th birthday this year. In June 2018, the current UK Prime Minister, Theresa May, highlighted that the NHS's £114bn budget would rise by an average of 3.4% annually. This is good news, but only if more money is being spent on well-being or lifestyle medicine. This is also supported by the NHS's England Five Year Forward plan, which highlights that the NHS needs to be financially sustainable, and it needs "a radical upgrade in prevention and public health."

This is where this book *Five-and-a-half ways to well-being* comes into the picture. The primary purpose of the book is to show that well-being is not some unattainable, foreign concept, and the book provides a solid grounding in why well-being is a powerful and effective concept. My aim is to guide you to unleash the alchemist dormant within you so that you can achieve your full potential, contribute to the world and live a fulfilling life.

By following these five-and-a-half ways to well-being, you will learn powerful, down-to-earth lifestyle medicine approaches for how you can become your own health coach!

To your health and wellness,
Ruben

# About the Author

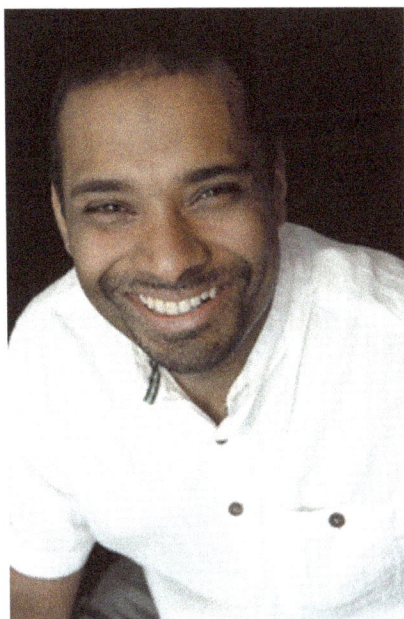

My name is Ruben Sherandra Seetharamdoo, or "Ruben," as my friends around the world know me. I am dedicated to helping you cut through the overly hyped diet, exercise and fitness nonsense that is running rampant in today's health and wellness industry. I am here to give you the in-depth information you've been seeking to get into the best shape of your life! I'll give you the benefit of my health and wellness expertise, so you'll soon be eating and exercising healthier than ever. My life's work revolves around seeking out tried and true, well-grounded principles for creating a foundation of total health and wellness. With your best interests in mind, I've applied my 15+ years of education and international experience in human psychology, science, health and wellness to provide you with a customised "toolkit-for-life"—one that you can live with and enjoy using every day of your life. This toolkit is packed to the brim with easy-to-understand concepts and doable techniques that will revitalise and rejuvenate your daily lifestyle. I promise that this toolkit will work to help you transform your quality of life and create the best mind/body fitness and vitality you've ever experienced. But first, here's a little about me and my background and why I am a health messenger.

## HOW I GREW UP.

I was born on the island of Mauritius. As a child, I started playing football at the tender age of just five years old. I immediately fell in love with the sport. Fast-forward several years and I realised my dream of playing for my school team at an amateur level! However, what I didn't tell you is that for 14 of those years, I equated fitness to health. The truth of the matter is: being physically fit is not always the same as being in good health. Even though I was involved in competitive sports, I did not have the best of health. At a very young age, I decided to become a vegetarian so that I could have optimal health. But being vegetarian alone is not good enough!

## I ALMOST HAD TO DIE FIRST!

As a matter of fact, I got into studying health, natural health sciences, well-being, and longevity in a very odd way. It's true! Back in 1997, while I was completing my first degree in chemistry, I had a near-death experience that really opened my eyes to just how important our health is and how much we often take it for granted. In 1997, I overcame a life-threatening bout of typhoid fever. This left me weak and listless for months. Then, a couple of months later, I had a severe bout of food poisoning and landed in the hospital. I experienced life-threatening complications while recovering from my bout of food poisoning, which actually caused my heart to stop! My life flashed before my eyes. I had a near-death experience and I was subjected to heart shock treatment with a defibrillator! The doctors told me that I was **very** lucky to be alive. Well, this incident really triggered something in me, and it was a great wake-up call regarding my health. Over the next several years, I dedicated much of my life to learning about health and wellness. I went on a mission to find all the best health, diet and wellness programs available. I spent thousands of pounds on all of the books, audio CDs, workshops, and custom training seminars on health, wellness, and longevity that I could find. I learned from top experts in health and wellness, like Deepak Chopra, Tony Robbins, Joseph McClendon, David Wolfe, Dr Colin Campbell and more. But it was **one** book in particular that had the most profound and life-changing effect on me. It was *The Alchemist* by Paulo Coelho—a book about becoming self-empowered, overcoming your mental blocks, and believing in your dreams.

And after I read it, I realised that everything in life is possible as long as you really want it to happen. But in my mind, all my dreams were dependent on my health. After all, if you aren't healthy, you won't be able to enjoy your life's dreams as much!

I transitioned from chemist to alchemist and published my first book on Amazon!

It made me want to follow my dream of helping as many people as I could to improve their own lives through better health and wellness. And for me, that meant I made the transition from a chemist to an alchemist! In fact, that book meant so much to me that I named my entire wellness company after it! My company name is "Unleash the Alchemist Within, Ltd".

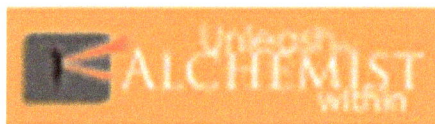

And all of this has led me to continually focus my energy and studies on cutting-edge health and wellness information. And it has actually helped me to become one of the foremost authorities in the field. I'm sharing this with you because I want you to know that I have what it takes to help you live at your absolute healthiest and best. Now let's get back to my story about how I became a world-renowned speaker, respected author, wellness consultant and scientist.

My first book is called *The Tried and Tested 12 Practical Steps Blueprint: How you can crush your addictive habits naturally and easily using cutting edge mind technology and the neurosciences in 21 days,* and it is available on Amazon. After I obtained my University degree, I had an overwhelming need to share what I had learned about health, physical and mental fitness, and enhanced wellness with others. My quest for knowledge led me to the Dale Carnegie's Institute where I did a 12-week leadership training to understand the true nuances of leadership. I continued my quest and attended university to complete my studies in psychiatric nursing. Being a registered mental health nurse gave me incredible insights into human behaviour, which I now use in my everyday life and my coaching and training methods. This opened a whole new world for me! I decided to finish my behavioural training and went on to complete my Master's degree with the Open University. I eventually completed my PhD, where my thesis was focused on addictive behaviour and the neurosciences. It was during this time in my life that I was introduced to neuro-linguistic programming (NLP) and NLP training. NLP became a source of incredible inspiration for my pursuit of the inner connection between the mind/body link and how to enable significant lifestyle changes. In 2008, I became a neuro-energetics certified trainer in neuro-linguistic programming and humanistic neuro-linguistic psychology during a four-week intensive residential training that I attended in Arizona in the United States. My expertise grew, and in order to become a certified NLP trainer, I carried on with my epistemological quest for knowledge and got a post-graduate coaching qualification from Oxford Brookes University. In my quest for evidence-based health coaching, I became interested in HeartMath and related health issues that deal with the interconnection of the mind, heart, and brain. In turn, this led me to dive even deeper into the science of wellness and patient recovery. In 2011, I became a licensed coach in HeartMath and emotional resilience. My work expertise ranged from working in Harley Street, the NHS, the Priory Hospital and internationally in the USA. My health and wellness experience has been extensive and varied. Over the years of my health and wellness career, I have worked in various disciplines of health in the National Health Service (NHS) in the UK, including oncology, learning disability, stoke, and palliative care. I was intrigued by this type of work, and I honed my clinical skills and used my expertise in private hospitals like the Priory Hospital in London. Later, I went even deeper into the most difficult to reach patients with substance misuse problems. In recent years, I worked in Massachusetts in the USA, where I helped young people with dual-diagnosis problems. All this led me to become a better health coach and allowed me to create my own coaching programmes. I've taught my optimal health and energy tips to so many others, and they gotten great results as well. Over the years, I've learned so many techniques about being healthier and improving all aspects of life. And, the more I learned, the more I realised I could help so many other people improve their health and overall happiness in their lives. The most amazing thing is: the more friends and family members I showed these techniques to, the more they worked like magic. Friends and family were losing weight, gaining strength and energy, and starting to tell me that they had never looked or felt this good before. Many friends kept telling me "Ruben you've GOT to teach this stuff to MORE people. You can help SO many other people out. And that's exactly what I've been doing ever since. I knew this needed to be available to more people, so I've put together a number of health and wellness workshops and retreats that you can now use to lose weight, get in shape, increase your strength and energy, improve your feelings of wellness and peace of mind, and got fantastic feedback!

I was voted Health Coach of the Year in the UK in March of 2013. My current forte is not only as a clinician and manager in the NHS but also as a health coach, scientist, author and speaker. I love training, coaching and consulting in health and wellness. As a fellow of the Royal Society of Public Health and having been awarded Health Coach of the Year, my consulting and training services are high in demand. The downside of one-on-one coaching is there is only so much of me to go around! With that thought in mind, I have created several health online training programmes and started to write books that can impact the lives of many people and can be enjoyed right in the comfort of one's own home. Presently, I live in Berkshire in the UK with my lovely wife, Samanta. Various experiences have brought challenges into my life—out of which, my philanthropic nature imbibed a sense of understanding of human beings. I like to listen, to absorb and to talk back in a remedial way by bridging each person to his or her lost soul and potential in life.

Finally, I have been asked the question why "five-and-a-half ways to well-being" and not "five ways to well-being," as everyone calls it? I am glad the question was asked, and the simple answer is "if you do what everyone else is doing, you will get the results everyone else is getting." Many people, including health professionals, have read about five ways of well-being and enjoyed it. Research says that less than ten percent of people put into practise what they read in self-help books. Consequently, this is why most people do not get any results. As a health coach, I want you to get great results in terms of your well-being, and for you to achieve this, you have to take action. That is why I have added a chapter to this book on "half way to well-being" to give you strategies to provide you with motivation and inspiration so that you can take massive action and, in turn, enable you to get massive results in terms of your health and well-being.

Please feel free to email me your success stories, feedback and suggestions about his book to ruben@ drrubenseetharamdoo.com.

Happy reading and enjoy the well-being adventure!

# TABLE OF CONTENTS

# 5 ½ WAYS

## — TO —

# WELL-BEING

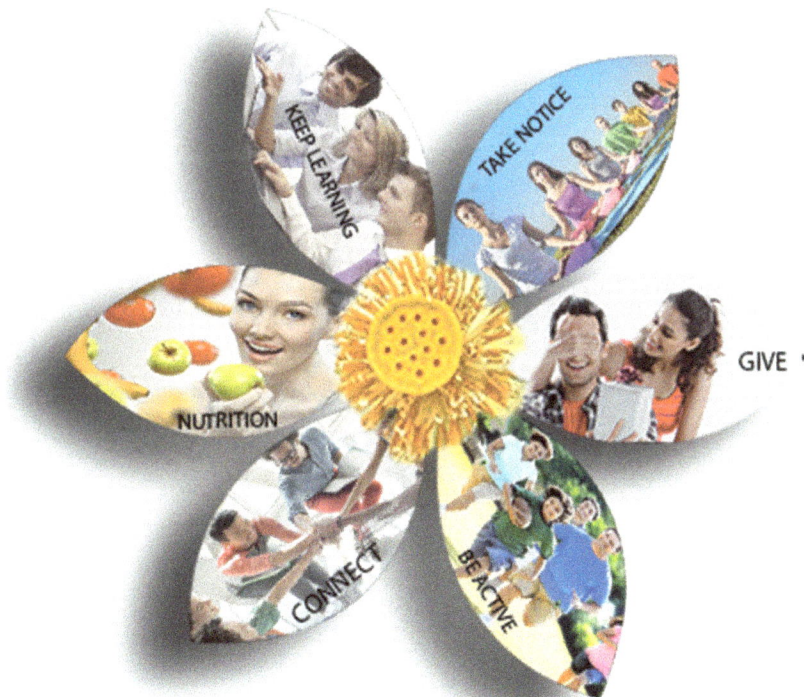

# Introduction

What if you could begin to transform your life so that you could increase your well-being starting right now? It wouldn't cost any money, and you don't need to break the bank for lifelong vitality and happiness. It wouldn't require any strenuous effort on your part. You could begin to do it from any place you happen to be. And you could go at your own pace.

Would you do it?

Would you even believe it's possible?

If you answered no, it wouldn't be surprising. Until the last few decades, the emphasis on mental health has been on psychological disorders, with very little study devoted to ordinary people increasing the fulfilment they can experience as they live their everyday lives.

All that has changed, and for some excellent reasons. It's now possible to scientifically measure happiness. And, even more surprising, there are tools that you and I, as ordinary people, can use to increase our "mental capital" or psychological and emotional well-being. These concepts have been proven time and again through scientific studies.

## THE POWER OF WELL-BEING

New research in the field known as positive psychology shows that we all have more control over our happiness than was previously thought, so there has been a shift in research to an investigation of how people can become happier by making changes in how they act and think.

Scientists have known for several decades that genetics are responsible for a large part of our temperament. By studying identical twins, research has determined that about 50% of our happiness (or unhappiness) can be traced to our genes. Another 10% is due to life circumstances such as marital status, our appearance, where we live, or how much money we have. The final 40% of our happiness is the result of what we think and what we do—and these things are choices. [1] Here's something that might surprise you. Did you know that what you think about can actually transform your brain? Studies have shown, for instance, that if a person sits quietly for a half-hour a day, thinking thoughts of kindness and compassion, their brain will show obvious changes in just two weeks. [2] Studies of Buddhist monks, subjects who deliberately and consistently cultivate positive emotions, show them registering happiness levels off the charts.

These findings are not "psycho-babble;" they're neuroscience. And they're so important that governments, such as that of Great Britain, and leaders throughout the world are choosing to fund research and create programs that concentrate on the happiness of their people.

## MYTHS ABOUT WELL-BEING

Is well-being just some foreign concept? Is well-being something that busy and intelligent people should not waste their precious time on? I have to admit that I am not a big fan of politics but when a politician is doing something good, I have to acknowledge it. Former British Prime Minister, David Cameron, has proven to be in the vanguard of those who support the concept of well-being as he speaks about "measuring our progress as a country not just by how our economy is growing, but by how our lives are improving…not just by our standard of living, but by our quality of life." He discusses the importance of making policy that supports people's feeling of being in control, being able to make choices, and having a sense of purpose and belonging.

Cameron addresses three concerns of the British public. (These might be on your mind as well, as you think about the concept of well-being.)

1. Is this concern with well-being a distraction from the major, urgent economic tasks at hand?

Cameron replied that "Growth is the essential foundation of all our aspirations . . . Our most urgent priority is to get the economy moving, to create jobs, to spread opportunity for everyone. But, if you know, both in your gut and from a huge body of evidence that prosperity alone can't deliver a better life, then you've got to take practical steps to make sure government is properly focused on our quality of life as well as economic growth, and that's what we're trying to do."

2. You can't really affect people's quality of life, so why try?

Cameron responded, "Just as we can create the climate for business to thrive, so we can create a climate in this country that is more family-friendly and more conducive to the good life. I would say that finding out what will really improve lives, and acting on it, is actually the serious business of government."

3. Isn't this well-being project a bit airy-fairy and impractical?

Cameron responded, "This information will help government work out, with evidence, the best ways of trying to help to improve people's well-being. This measure we are setting up today will open a national debate about how together we can build a better life. It will lead to government policy that is more focused not just on the bottom line, but on all those things that make life worthwhile." [3]

## THE WORLDWIDE TREND

The United Nations has recognised March 20th as the International Day of Happiness, a day for celebrating and reflecting on happiness. This is a serious move in which the UN encourages us to be responsible and work through difficulties rather than assigning blame to others. It has commissioned reports such as the World Happiness Report of 2012, in which the reasons for happiness in 152 countries have been studied.

The World Happiness Report combines the talents of three distinguished experts:

- Richard Layard, director of the well-being programme at the London

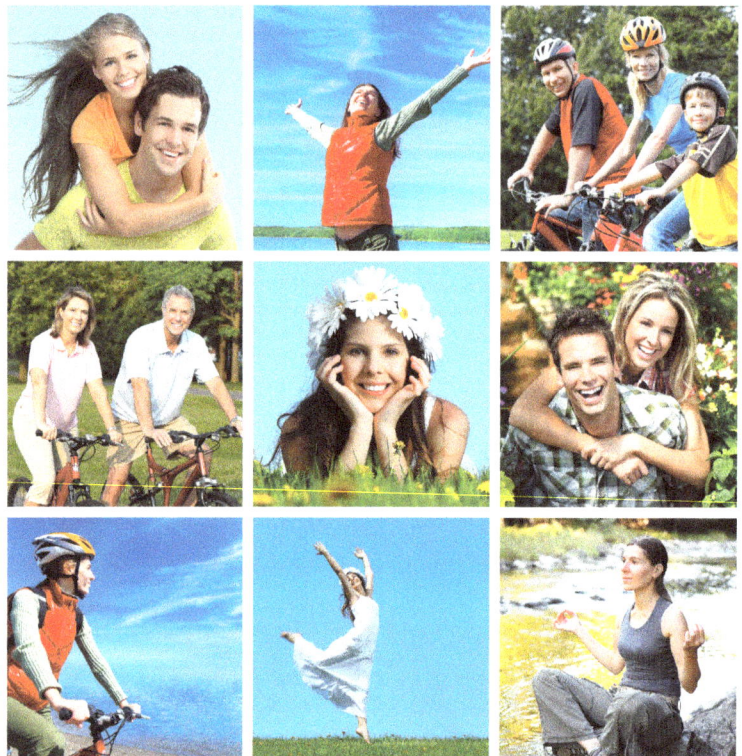

School of Economics' Centre for Economic Performance, and author of the book *Happiness—Lessons from a New Science.*
- John Helliwell, of the Economics Department of the University of British Columbia and co-director of the "Social Interactions, Identity and Well-being" program of the Canadian Institute for Advanced Research.
- Jeffrey D. Sachs, director of The Earth Institute, and professor of Health Policy and Management at Columbia University.[4] In creating this report, these gentlemen were concerned with accurately measuring people's happiness within and across societies, and whether these measurements could be used to provide valid information to guide policymaking. The report concludes that regular collection of happiness data on a large scale will enable analysis of policies on well-being, which will improve macroeconomic policymaking.

The report discusses the causes of happiness and misery, based on 30 years of research. It discusses external and personal aspects. External factors include income, work, community and governance, and values and religion. Personal factors include mental and physical health, family experience, education, gender, and age and how there can be a two-way interaction between these factors. The analysis shows that while absolute income is important, especially in poor countries, many other variables have a more powerful effect on happiness—among these are social trust, quality of work, and freedom of choice and political participation. [5]

The report's conclusions are based on the research of sociologists and psychologists observing concrete factors' impact on happiness. Gross National Product (GNP) is only one of many factors; others are inequalities, extreme poverty, ill health, and many more. The report concludes that beyond health, economic, and societal influences, happiness depends primarily on the lifestyle we adopt—and "We can improve our quality of life by adopting a lifestyle and technologies that enhance happiness or well-being."

The UN advocates that each one of us:

- Confronts what hampers the development of our happiness.
- Engages in a responsible lifestyle.
- Uses appropriate technologies to help us with the process. [6]

This approach to well-being takes into account not only the scientific breakthroughs of the last couple of decades but also the widespread use of technology even in poorer countries, and the many benefits technology can offer people.

## WHAT IS WELL-BEING?

"Well-being is a dynamic state in which the individual is able to develop their potential, work productively and creatively, build strong and positive relationships with others, and contribute to their community. It is enhanced when an individual is able to fulfil their personal and social goals and achieve a sense of purpose in society." [7]

### The Foresight Project: The Mental Capital and Well-Being Project

The Foresight Project involved over 400 experts and included over 100 commissioned reviews of the state of the science of well-being. According to well-being experts, well-being is how people experience their lives rather than the objective facts of their lives. It's possible for a person to have a sense of well-being even though their circumstances might not be favourable. It is also possible for a person in very favourable circumstances to feel his or her life is empty or stagnant.[8]

According to research, a high level of well-being is associated with positive functioning, which includes creative thinking, productivity, good interpersonal relationships and resilience in the face of adversity, along with good physical health and good life expectancy. This person experiences frequent positive emotions, positive attitudes toward himself, others, and events, and positive behaviours such as setting and achieving goals or pursuing a healthy lifestyle.

A low level of well-being is associated with less positive functioning and a lower level of health and life expectancy. These (people on this level) are the people who could benefit from strategies to improve their well-being.[9]

To put this in perspective, the Warwick-Edinburgh Mental Well-being Scale (WEMWBS) divides the population into four segments: flourishing, moderate mental health, languishing, and mental disorder. Not all statistics are available in the UK, but it is estimated that at any time one-sixth or 17% of the population has some form of mental health problem.[10] US statistics show 11% as languishing, 55% as having moderate mental health, and 17% as flourishing.[11] These statistics indicate two critical points:

- 66% of the population (those languishing and those with moderate mental health) could directly benefit from strategies to improve well-being.
- Shifting the mean (the number of people languishing and with moderate mental health) could have a dramatic impact on decreasing the number of people with mental disorders and on increasing the number of those who flourish.[12]

Evidence shows that this level of well-being can be changed as a result of various types of learning or training.[13]

The Foresight Project concluded that "Strengthening individuals (with a low level of well-being) could be accomplished through practises designed to promote self-efficacy; emotional/social skills and resilience; intrinsic motivation and sense of purpose; empathy and prosocial behaviour; and lifestyles that enhance and protect mental health, such as physical activity, nutrition, drinking moderately, and maintain social networks."[14]

## 5 WAYS TO WELL-BEING

The Foresight Project commissioned the centre for well-being at the NEF (the New Economics Foundation) to create a set of actions based on Foresight's findings on well-being. The NEF, whose mission is "economics as if people and the planet mattered," aimed to develop a generic set of actions based on evidence that would enhance individual personal well-being for a wide range of people. This set of actions became *Five Ways to Well-being*.

## 5 AND ½ WAYS TO WELL-BEING

The scientific evidence revealed five areas where specific behaviour could enhance well-being: social relationships, physical activity, awareness, learning, and giving. NEF organised these into five key actions:

- Connect: Connecting with your family, friends, colleagues and neighbours to support and enrich you every day.
- Be Active: Finding an activity you enjoy and taking part in it on most days to increase your mental and physical well-being.

- Take Notice: Noticing what's happening around you and experiencing it along with your own thoughts and feelings gives you an increased awareness of life and appreciation for it.
- Keep Learning: Learning new skills gives you a sense of achievement and increases your self-confidence. And it can be great fun, too.
- Give to others: Whether it's small things or larger ones, whether it's giving to friends or strangers, it's rewarding and increases your sense of well-being.

Those are the five steps that, if taken, have been scientifically proven to increase well-being. They might surprise you. You might have expected other factors like income to play a more significant part. You'll probably agree that each one of these steps can be taken by each one of us if we choose to do so. [15]

And now I'm sure you're wondering about the ½ step. Maybe you've guessed by now. Let me give you a hint: What very often gets in the way of us succeeding in the things we take on? That's right, you've guessed it. We lose interest. We drop out. We stop doing the activity. We quit. So much promise; so little reward.

In the remaining chapters of this ebook, we'll discuss many ways to accomplish these steps to well-being and explore ways to remain motivated so that we achieve the well-being we desire.

## WELL-BEING SELF-ASSESSMENT TEST

Mental well-being is not just the absence of mental problems. It's about feeling good and functioning well in your life. Really, it's about having the ability to experience your life in a complete and positive way and enjoy it.

As interest in well-being increases, people and governments alike are more interested in individuals being able to assess their own well-being. Online, self-reporting tests are being developed which will measure objective well-being with validity. For instance, the BBC-SWB scale, which measured well-being in 23,3431 participants, is considered "a reliable and valid measure for the online assessment of subjective well-being in the general population." [16]

The questionnaire below uses WEMWBS (The Warwick-Edinburgh Mental Well-being Scale) to measure mental well-being. It was created by mental well-being experts and has been used by scientists and psychologists worldwide since 2007. [17]

To get your own well-being score, go through the following statements and tick the box that best describes your thoughts and feelings over the last two weeks.

**QUESTIONS**

1. I've been feeling optimistic about the future
   a) None of the time (1 point)
   b) Rarely (2 points)
   c) Some of the time (3 points)
   d) Often (4 points)
   e) All of the time (5 points)

2. I've been feeling useful
   a) None of the time (1 point)
   b) Rarely (2 points)
   c) Some of the time (3 points)
   d) Often (4 points)
   e) All of the time (5 points)

3. I've been feeling relaxed
   a) None of the time (1 point)
   b) Rarely (2 points)
   c) Some of the time (3 points)
   d) Often (4 points)
   e) All of the time (5 points)

4. I've been feeling interested in other people
   a) None of the time (1 point)
   b) Rarely (2 points)
   c) Some of the time (3 points)
   d) Often (4 points)
   e) All of the time (5 points)

5. I've had energy to spare
   a) None of the time (1 point)
   b) Rarely (2 points)
   c) Some of the time (3 points)
   d) Often (4 points)
   e) All of the time (5 points)

6. I've been dealing with problems well
   a) None of the time (1 point)
   b) Rarely (2 points)
   c) Some of the time (3 points)
   d) Often (4 points)
   e) All of the time (5 points)

7. I've been thinking clearly
   a) None of the time (1 point)
   b) Rarely (2 points)
   c) Some of the time (3 points)
   d) Often (4 points)
   e) All of the time (5 points)

8. I've been feeling good about myself
   a) None of the time (1 point)
   b) Rarely (2 points)
   c) Some of the time (3 points)
   d) Often (4 points)
   e) All of the time (5 points)

9. I've been feeling close to other people
   a) None of the time (1 point)
   b) Rarely (2 points)
   c) Some of the time (3 points)
   d) Often (4 points)
   e) All of the time (5 points)

10. I've been feeling confident
    a) None of the time (1 point)
    b) Rarely (2 points)
    c) Some of the time (3 points)
    d) Often (4 points)
    e) All of the time (5 points)

11. I've been able to make up my own mind about things
    a) None of the time (1 point)
    b) Rarely (2 points)
    c) Some of the time (3 points)
    d) Often (4 points)
    e) All of the time (5 points)

12. I've been feeling loved
    a) None of the time (1 point)
    b) Rarely (2 points)
    c) Some of the time (3 points)
    d) Often (4 points)
    e) All of the time (5 points)

13. I've been interested in new things
    a) None of the time (1 point)
    b) Rarely (2 points)
    c) Some of the time (3 points)
    d) Often (4 points)
    e) All of the time (5 points)

14. I've been feeling cheerful
    a) None of the time (1 point)
    b) Rarely (2 points)
    c) Some of the time (3 points)
    d) Often (4 points)
    e) All of the time (5 points)

## RESULTS

0-32 points

Your well-being score is very low. Most people have a score between 41 and 59. You may want to begin by talking to a friend or health professional about how you can start to address this. There are five evidence-based steps we can all take to improve our mental well-being. They are:

- Get active
- Connect with others

- Keep learning
- Be aware of yourself and the world

Give to others. Go to useful links for more on the five steps.

## 32-40 points

Your well-being score is below average. Most people have a score between 41 and 59. Why not take action to improve your mental well-being?

There are five evidence-based steps we can all take to improve our mental well-being. They are:

- Get active
- Connect with others
- Keep learning
- Be aware of yourself and the world

Give to others Go to useful links for more on the five steps.

## 40-59 points

Your well-being score is average. Most people have a score between 41 and 59. You can still improve your mental well-being by taking action. There are five evidence-based steps we can all take to improve our mental well-being. They are:

- Get active
- Connect with others
- Keep learning
- Be aware of yourself and the world
- Give to others

## 59-70 points

Good news, your well-being score is above average. Most people have a score between 41 and 59. Continue doing the things that are keeping you happy.

(Source:http://www.nhs.uk/Tools/Pages/Wellbeing-self-assessment.aspx)[18]

How did you do? Don't worry if your score isn't as high as you might like. If you follow the suggestions in this book, you'll be on your way to increased well-being for the rest of your life.

# CONNECT

*"The most basic and powerful way to connect to another person is to listen. Just listen. Perhaps the most important thing we ever give each other is our attention.... A loving silence often has far more power to heal and to connect than the most well-intentioned words."*
— Rachel Naomi Remen

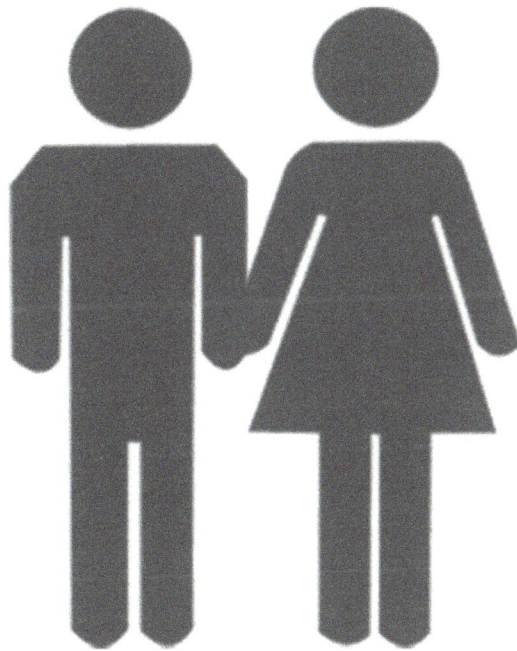

# HAVE YOU HEARD ABOUT THE ROSETO EFFECT?

You might be asking what the Roseto effect has to do with connecting? Well, the Roseto effect is the phenomenon by which a close-knit community experiences a reduced rate of heart disease. The effect is named after a little town called Roseto, located in eastern Pennsylvania. From 1954 to 1961, Roseto had nearly no heart attacks for the otherwise high-risk group of men 55 to 64. An analysis of public health data concluded that Roseto was a very healthy place to live, but no one could find out the reasons why. As a result, researchers went to Roseto to investigate and stayed for several years.

Initial findings by investigators were mind-boggling. They found out that the Rosetans smoked cigars, drank copious amount of alcohol and skipped the Mediterranean diet in favour of sausages fried in lard with cheeses. The men did not have any office jobs but worked in the slate quarries in very toxic environmental conditions. However, Roseto was found to have no crime rates and a very low number of requests for police assistance.

So, what made Rosetans die less from heart disease than neighbouring towns, like Bangor in Pennsylvania? The answer from extensive research: They had traditional and cohesive family and community relationships. It turns out that Roseto was populated by tight-knit Italian-American families who did most things together. In a nutshell, Rosetans were nourished by people.

However, a decade or so later as Roseto became more Americanised and the inhabitants become increasingly isolated, the rates of heart disease has become identical to other towns in Pennsylvania.

In the book, *The Power of Clan*, the authors who covered the town of Roseto from 1935-1984 concluded that: "The magic of Roseto was because Rosetans didn't feel isolated or crushed, rather they avoided the internalisation of stress. Stability and predictability...hardly Americanised virtues...even in the early years, was life soothing; hence life lengthening."

For me, the Roseto effect illustrates the big "why" we need to connect for well-being.

# CONNECTION WITH HUMAN BEINGS

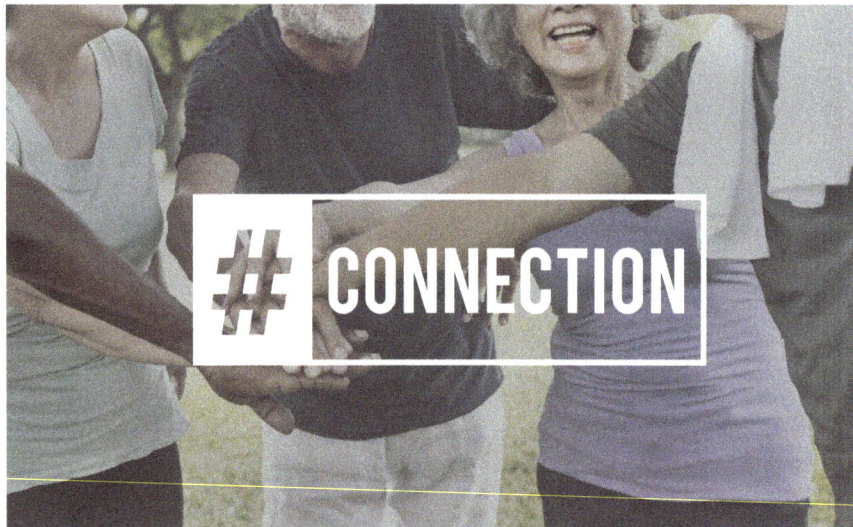

Connect. . .

"With the people around you. With family, friends, colleagues and neighbours. At home, work, school or in your local community. Think of these as the cornerstones of your life and invest time into developing them. Building these connections will support and enrich you every day." [19]

The Forsyth Challenge Reports indicated that social relationships are critical for promoting well-being.

Our social relationships act as buffers for us at any age and seemed to protect against mental ill health. In fact, surveys conducted in Great Britain on adults between the ages of 16 to 64 reveal that the main difference between people with mental disorders and those without them is social participation. [20]

Interestingly, data from the 2005 British Attitude Survey shows that since 1989, there's been an increase with both men and women in the number of people who would rather spend more time with family and friends and less time at work.[21] Several studies indicate that life goals associated with commitment to family and friends promote life satisfaction, while life goals associated with career success and material gain are detrimental to life satisfaction.[22] So, real-life preferences about social communication and studies about the effects of social communication support each other.

A person can have two kinds of relationships: Broad social network relationships with lots of people, and strong, deeper, more supportive and meaningful relationships with a few people. Both types are essential for well-being since broad relationships create a sense of connectedness, while strong relationships provide a sense of support. [23]

## It Starts With You

There's no getting around it. The quality of all your relationships begins with you. You are at the core. You are the heart and soul. What you put in is very much what you get out. Is that stating the obvious? Well, yes and no. You see, there's probably no area in our lives fraught with more deception than how we see ourselves. Let me illustrate.

Have you heard of Brene Brown? She's a PhD, LMSW writer and research professor at the University of Houston Graduate College of Social Work in the United States. She's been featured prominently, with appearances on CNN, the TED talks, and the Oprah Winfrey show, as well as many other places.

So, this sounds like a woman who might have an understanding of who she is, right? Well, that's what she thought, too. In her book, *The Gifts of Imperfection: Let Go of Who You Think You're Supposed to Be and Embrace Who You Are (Your Guide to a Wholehearted Life)*, she gives us a clear account of just how wrong she was about that.

Here's her story. She begins by telling us that, as a researcher, her job is to observe human behaviour and identify, "The subtle connections, relationships, and patterns that help us make meaning of our thoughts, behaviours, and feelings." [24]

Her job consisted of analysing data and making sense of it. In the study she was doing in November of 2006, she was trying to define what it meant to live "wholeheartedly" by studying a group of people who clearly lived that way. These participants trusted themselves and talked about authenticity and love and belonging in a way she didn't completely understand. She wanted to know:

- What did these folks value?
- How did they become so resilient?
- What were their main concerns?
- How did they resolve or address those concerns?
- Can anyone create this wholehearted life they have?
- What does it take to cultivate what we need to do it?
- What gets in the way? [25]

Brene decided to divide her data into two columns, the Do's and Don'ts. At the end of her process, the Do column was filled with words like worthiness, rest, play, trust, faith, intuition, hope, authenticity, love, belonging, joy, gratitude, and creativity. The Don't column held words like perfection, numbing, certainty, exhaustion, self-sufficiency, being cool, fitting in, judgment, and scarcity. [26]

(Just out of curiosity, which column describes you?)

As she looked at the lists, Brene received quite a shock. She fully expected to find herself in the Do column, with the Wholehearted people behaving exactly as she did: working hard, following the rules, persisting until she got it right, raising her kids by the book, ceaselessly trying to understand herself better, and so on. [27]

What she learned that day was that she was getting it wrong. In her words,

"How much we know and understand ourselves is critically important, but there is something that is even more essential to living a Wholehearted life: loving ourselves."

"Knowledge is important, but only if we're being kind and gentle with ourselves as we work to discover who we are. Wholeheartedness is as much about embracing our tenderness and vulnerability as it is about developing knowledge and claiming power." [28]

It became obvious to Brene that the real journey was equally heart work and head work, and she was failing the heart work. She was so busy trying to live up to who she thought she was supposed to be, she had next to no idea of who she really was.

That's a fairly common state for us as human beings even though the universe regularly gives us situations to help us uncover who we really are. Over the course of our lives, most of us experience many of these challenges:

- Marriage.
- Divorce
- Middle-age.
- Becoming a parent.
- Retirement.
- Loss of trauma.
- Serious illness or injury.
- Working in a job we hate.

But, as Brene puts it, "The universe is not short on wake-up calls. We're just quick to hit the snooze button." Still, she's adamant that the results are worth the messy, sometimes difficult journey of facing ourselves as we really are. If you choose to do the work of getting to know your authentic self, what happened to her will happen for you as well. She describes it this way:

"Oh, my God. I feel different. I feel joyful. I'm still afraid, but I also feel really brave. Something has changed—I can feel it in my bones." [29]

"I was healthier, more joyful, and more grateful than I had ever felt. I felt calmer and grounded, and significantly less anxious. I had rekindled my creative life, reconnected with my family and friends in a new way, and most important felt truly comfortable in my own skin for the first time in my life. I was setting new boundaries and began to let go of my need to please, perform, and perfect." [30]

These statements capture the essence of living out the Five Ways to Well-being program:

"I now see how owning our story and loving ourselves through that process is the bravest thing that we will ever do."

"I now see that courage, compassion, and connection only work when they are exercised. Every day."

"Owning our story can be hard but not nearly as difficult as spending our lives running from it. Embracing our vulnerabilities is risky, but not nearly as dangerous as giving up on love and belonging and joy—the experiences that make us the most vulnerable. Only when we are brave enough to explore the darkness will we discover the infinite power of our light." [31]

A real connection with others is a choice you make again and again on a daily basis. It's a choice that is vital to your own well-being.

## The Importance Of Friends And Family

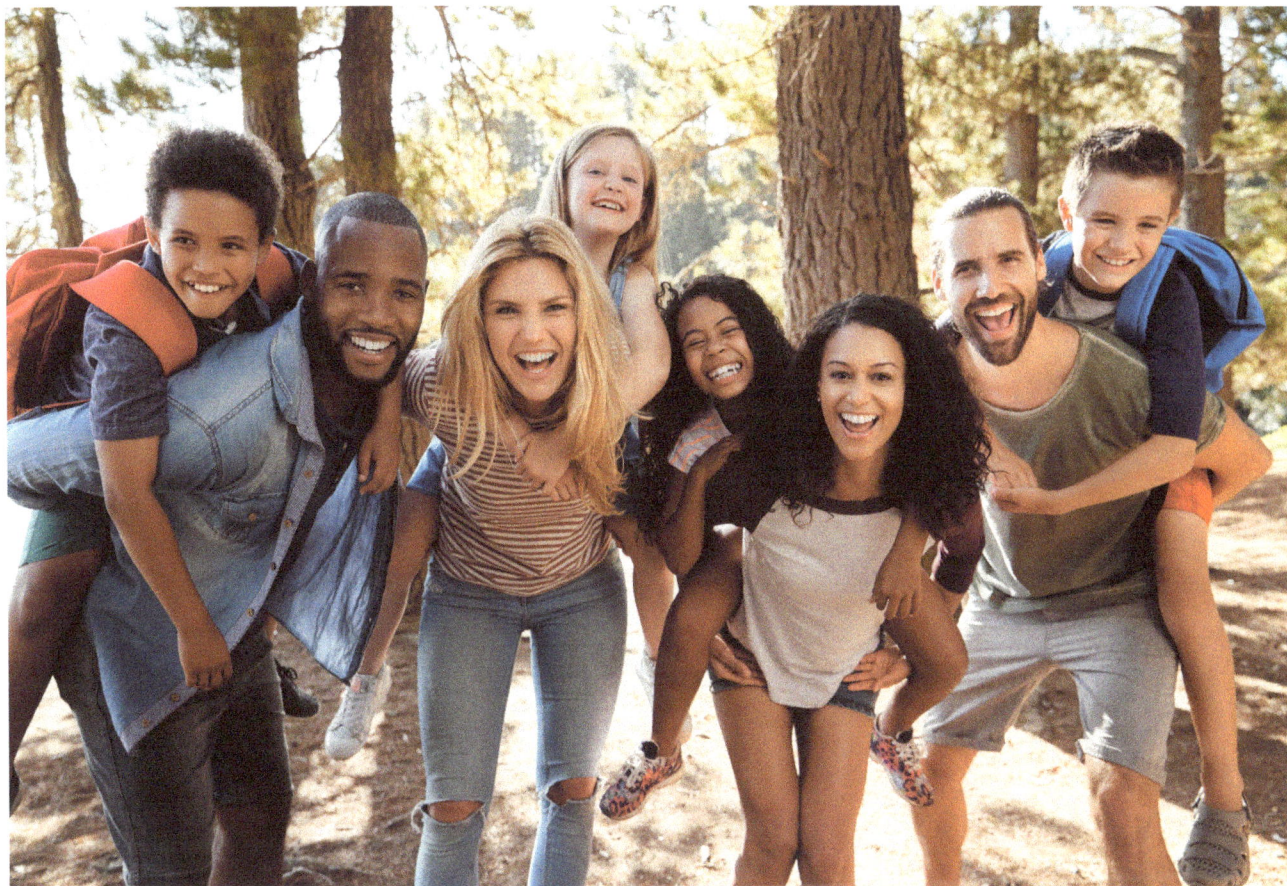

Healthy relationships—whether with friends, family, colleagues or others—are a critical component of health and well-being. Scientific evidence supports the theory that strong relationships contribute to a long, healthy, happy life while being isolated or alone in life is as great a risk factor as smoking, high blood pressure, or obesity.

Findings from 148 studies revealed that people with strong social relationships are 50% less likely to die prematurely. In another study of over 100 people, it was found that participants completing a stressful task recovered faster when they were reminded of people with whom they had strong relationships. In yet another study, it was found that people who had strong relationships were half as likely to catch a common cold when exposed to the virus. [32]

On the other hand, a lack of social support had just the opposite effect. A 2012 study of breast cancer patients found that those who had fewer strong relationships suffered higher levels of depression, pain, and fatigue. The same study found a strong correlation between loneliness and decreased immune system function. That means that a lack of social connection can increase your risk of becoming sick. Another study at the University of Chicago followed 229 adults over five years. It found that loneliness correlated with higher incidences of high blood pressure. The conclusion is inevitable from these studies: the lack of relationships can cause problems with physical, emotional, and even spiritual well-being. [33]

So, how exactly can friends and family help you? First, anything you want to do that requires some effort and dedication can be easier with the encouragement of the people closest to you. They can motivate you, remind you of your goals, and give you positive feedback and encouragement.

Think about it. How much could you really accomplish as one isolated individual? Honestly, not much.

And that's true for all of us. Our positive relationships help us through hard times with understanding and solace and through everyday activities with advice, encouragement, and companionship.

Here are a few tips you can keep in mind that will help you build strong relationships day by day:

1. Communicate your feelings: let your friends and family know how you feel. This is how they get to know who you really are. Some people are easier to tell your feelings to than others, but if you express what you're feeling in an appropriate, non-threatening way, you'll increase your chances of being heard. Now, you may know people—even close family and friends—who simply will not hear you. But you probably know who those people are already.

2. Listen: people love to be heard. When you give others your full attention and listen to them with an open mind, you show that you respect them and care about them. Have you ever tried to tell somebody something but felt that the person had already made up their mind about you and what you had to say? It's not a good feeling, is it? You feel invisible and unimportant. On the other hand, when you pay full attention to the people you care about, you build trust and comfort with them.

3. Be vulnerable: yes, it isn't always easy to open up to other people, but if you don't, how can you form a trusting relationship? People can't get really close to you if they don't know the person under the mask. Being vulnerable means being brave. First, you're brave enough to take the mask off to yourself, so that you know who you really are. Second, you're brave enough to show your authentic self to the people you want to have deep relationships with.

4. Build trust: isn't trust what it's all about? Don't we all want a relationship where we feel safe, not judged, not betrayed, and not abandoned? A relationship where we can be truly ourselves? We can't have any of those things without trust. The way to build trust is to be open about your thoughts and feelings and to be supportive of the other person's.

5. Don't stereotype: there are all kinds of stereotypes based on gender, age, and other things ("Oh well, he's a guy!" or "She's too old!"). We've all heard statements like these, but these statements deny the individuality of the other person and reduce that person to a stereotype. Again, it's not seeing that person for who he or she really is. Take the time to recognise the other person's uniqueness if you want to build strong relationships.

6. Manage conflict: some disagreement is probably inevitable from time to time within all relationships. You should be able to feel and express your anger when it's warranted. But you should express anger in a fair, balanced way and focus on the issue rather than blaming or shaming the other person. This approach can lead to better communication, mutual respect, and successful problem-solving.

According to Bridget Granville-Cleave, a founding member of the International Positive Psychology Foundation in Britain and author of *Introducing Positive Psychology: A Practical Guide,* you have the ability to increase your happiness fivefold by the way you interact in your relationships. Here's what she says:

- The desire for connection is a fundamental human need.
- Your relationships (with family, friends, loved ones, colleagues and others) are a central source of well-being.
- People with strong, happy relationships experience five times more positive emotion than negative emotion.
- You can increase the positive emotion or reduce the negative emotion in your relationship to achieve the 5:1 positivity ratio. [34]

Now it's up to you. You know the science, and you have the knowledge to make it work. Will you make an effort to build positive relationships?

## Community

As human beings, we are social creatures, and we live in a community. Just as our individual health and well-being are tied to a connection with friends and family, is also tied up with our interactions with others outside our closest circle and interactions within our communities. Much of our behaviour is established by the community.

Many of our norms and habits may be at least partially established through our social networks. For instance, if several of your friends are smokers, you may believe that it's all right for you to smoke as well. Think of the 1950s, a time when medical science had not yet determined the health risks of smoking. Social norms told us that it was perfectly fine to smoke, even "cool."

Our social networks may influence us, but we can also influence them. We accomplish through social networks things we can't accomplish on our own. Because we are part of the community, we reap many benefits. Because we are a part of a community, we have access to many services such as schools and hospitals, the fire department and the police department, to name just a few. We may take these things for granted, or we may object to the taxes we pay to maintain them, but we all benefit.

A 2009 study by Helliwell and Putnam confirms that our subjective well-being is directly linked to the well-being of the community, and the well-being of the community is related to our individual happiness and life satisfaction.[35]

So, we benefit from our community because of the services we can access and the general well-being the healthy community offers. And there's a third, very important way we can benefit from our community; when we contribute our time and effort to our community, we derive a heightened sense of well-being. You can think of it as a sense of altruism or a sense of purpose, but however you see it, contributing to our community increases our self-esteem and confidence, and gives us a sense of greater control over our lives. Not only do we see ourselves in a more positive, charitable light, but we actually perceive others to be that way as well. Our focus shifts from the negativity of our own problems, and we create gratitude for the good things we do have.[36]

## Connecting With The Higher Power

The concept of connecting with one's higher power can be quite controversial for many. But again, if we have a look at the literature, there is a lot of evidence that this approach well very well for some people. Project Match is a good example that shows the effectiveness of 12 steps programs and how many people can restore their sanity by connecting to higher power.[36] My personal experience working with hundreds of individuals who attend mutual help groups is that they really benefited positively in their recovery by embracing the concept of higher power.

What is higher power after all? Higher power is a concept that has been coined in the 1930s and basically means a power that is greater than ourselves. A higher power can be anyone, for example, a Supreme Being, deity or God. The way different people connect with their higher power varies. Examples are meditating, reciting prayers.

One of my ways of connecting with my higher power is by the serenity prayer below:

"God, grant me the serenity to accept the things I cannot change,

The courage to change the things I can,

And wisdom to know the difference."

My question for you is as follows: Who is your higher power? And if you were to connect with your higher power, what will that look like? A prayer, meditation. . . Be open-minded, let go of the scepticism and give it a go!

## Connecting via the Worldwide Web/Social Networking

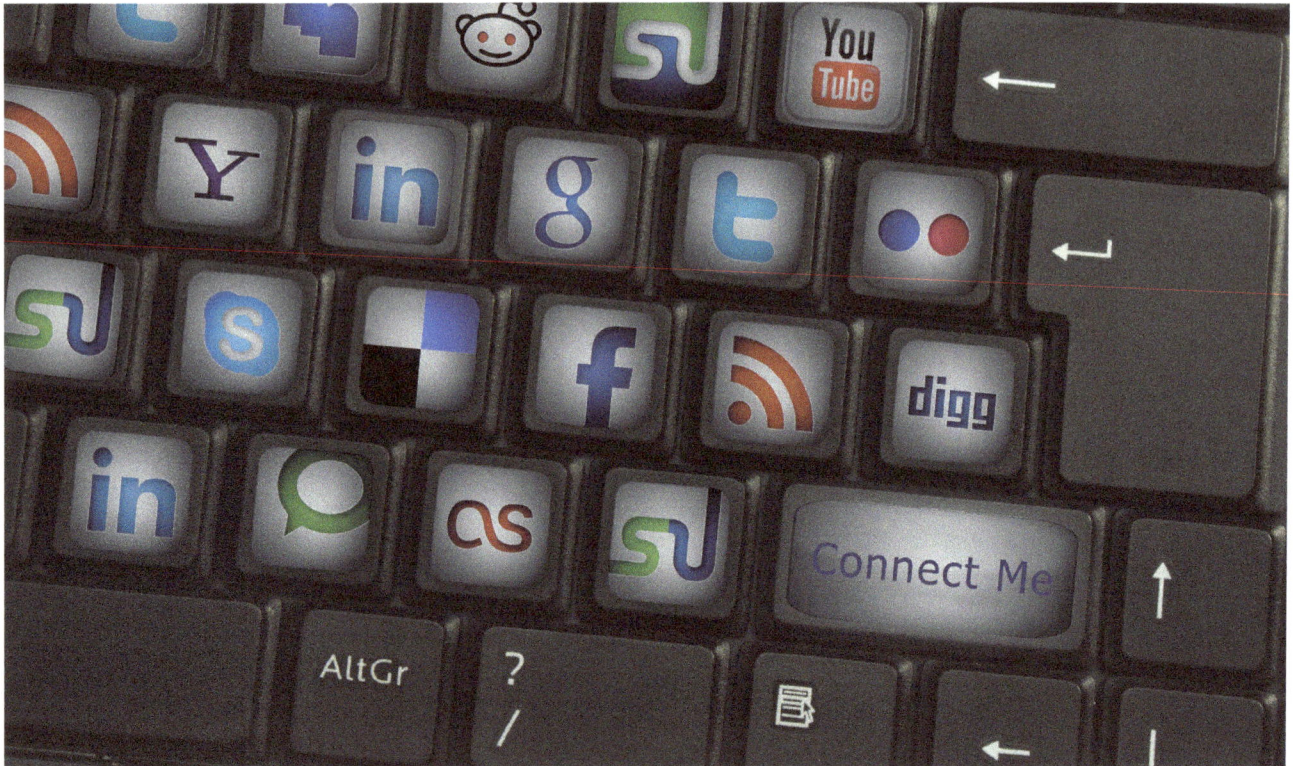

I like Brene Brown's definition of connection:

"Connection is the energy that exists between people when they feel seen, heard, and valued; when they can give and receive without judgment; and when they derive sustenance and strength from the relationship."

Neuroscience has shown that we are absolutely wired for connection. From the time we are born, we need it to thrive in every way—physically, emotionally, intellectually, and spiritually. We now understand that our relationships, along with our experiences, shape our personalities and that our relationships even impact the way our brain develops and performs. [37]

So, how confusing is it to be so connected to Facebook and Twitter and yet not necessarily seen or heard at all? How many of us, or people we know, spend much more time on social media where we are not face-to-face with anyone? How many times do we see people at "social" gatherings who are socialising with people on the other end of their smartphones? The question really is, "What is the effect of this on our well-being?"

The internet and social media give a whole new definition and intensity to the term "connecting," don't they?

The Internet is an amazing thing. It allows the free exchange of information across borders and without boundaries. It's undoubtedly changed life for the better by providing boundless knowledge and connectivity.

We can talk to people on the other side of the world with the greatest ease. We can locate long-lost friends and make new ones. Twitter users tweet 400 million times a day, while Facebook processes over 500 terabytes of new data every single day.[38] Access to information can be overwhelming, and so can access to banality—and that could be a problem.

Connection is so easy that it's a part of our lives that we take for granted now. Yet, we have to ask, "What is the quality of the time we're spending, and how is it affecting our well-being?"

Recent research is showing that connection via social media can have an adverse effect on our levels of happiness. This can happen in two ways: First, we spent a lot of time looking at idealised profiles of other people, which can make us feel inadequate with the reality of our own life. Second, we're bombarded by images of people who have more things and better things than we do, and we feel we have to keep up.

Psychologists have a term for this: the hedonic treadmill. It works like this: We go out and buy whatever we feel we have to have. The problem is that the satisfaction wears off in a few days. It never lasts. Eventually, we return to the buying treadmill once again. This cycle is true with comparing purchases and also with experiences. The satisfaction is never permanent.[39]

Think about experiences you've had or purchases you've made. Have you experienced the hedonic treadmill experience in your life?

Maybe the lesson here is one of balance. The internet can be used to enhance your well-being or leave you feeling a little empty and frustrated. It's up to you and how you use it.

And, one other thing while we're speaking of balance; remember that this program is about increasing your well-being. Not everyone you encounter will be a positive experience. It could be a stranger, a co-worker, or even a family member, but if someone in your life consistently treats you badly with criticism or in any other way, it's up to you to have your own best interests in mind. Give your time, attention, and energy to others with positive intentions like yours.

A word of warning about connecting with people:

Remember that for you to thrive in life, you need to connect with individuals who support you and challenge constructively. In fact, according to research from Michigan Business School, people you connect should use positive comments a lot more—about six times more—than criticism. If the reverse is true, you definitely need to evaluate your relationship with that person.

## What is Hoʻoponopono?

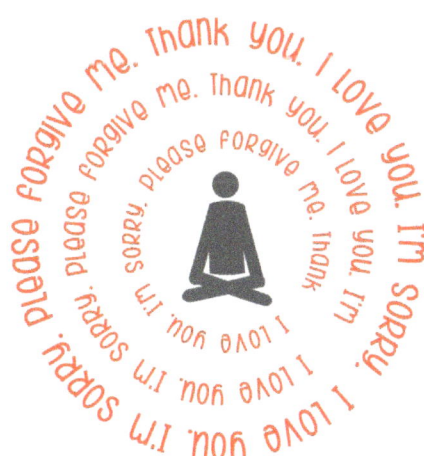

As we connect with human beings, we are sometimes bound to have misunderstandings, disagreements and arguments. In turn, these can lead us to harbour negative emotions such as anger, guilt, resentment towards one another. If we want lifelong vitality, optimal health and happiness, we have to forgive and let go of those negative emotions. This is easier said than done. This is the reason I want to introduce you to a very powerful technique that I have been teaching successfully to hundreds of my coachees as part of the humanistic neuro-linguisticpPsychology workshops I have been running. The technique is called: **Hoʻoponopono** (ho-o-pono-pono). This is a concept of ancient Hawaii, and it basically means "to make our relationships with everyone right."

This is an imagination exercise, and Einstein highlights that imagination is more powerful than knowledge. The steps you need to follow are as follows:

1. In your imagination, imagine a beautiful stage (It could be somewhere in nature, a stage in your favourite theatre.)
2. Invite the person who you don't have a good relationship with or connection with to come to the stage

3. Imagine in your mind's eye that you are connected with that person with an imaginary string or thread and have a conversation with the person and say the following mantra "I am sorry, please forgive me, I love you and I thank you",

4. In the spirit of Ho'oponopono, we all have another chance and opportunity to repair any damage and repeat to the other person "I am doing my part, and for the sake of all of us, I hope that you will do the same"

5. Eventually, imagine you take out your special pair of scissors and cut the imaginary string or thread that connect you to the other person

6. Just notice how you feel and from your heart imagine radiating pink love energy to the other person as you connect in a very new way.

This process takes only five minutes, and you can repeat the process with as many people as you wish.

## CONNECTION WITH NATURE

A human being is constantly aware of the influence of nature in the form of the earth they walk upon, the air they breathe, the water they drink, warmth from the sun and the surroundings in which they live.

### Connection with the Earth: Earthing

Connection with the Earth: Earthing

Have you heard about "earthing"? Earthing is a simple and natural process. Our human body—which is 80 percent water—is a natural conductor of electricity. When the human body has direct contact with the surface of the earth, free electrons from the earth are transferred to the human body, and this has been proven to have powerful antioxidants effects which are priceless for well-being. Therefore, earthing refers to the process of drawing from the Earth's energy by being in close contact with the Earth. You sit, stand, or walk on conductive surfaces—grass, sand or earth for half an hour and see if you notice whether your pain or stress diminishes. You could also experience it as a warm, pleasant tingling sensation, or as feeling better or having more energy than usual, or as sleeping very well—it's the beneficial effect of connection with the earth's energy.

Does that strike you as a little strange? Well, think about it for a minute. We as human beings have walked barefoot and slept on the earth throughout history. It's only been in modern times that we wear rubber-soled shoes that separate us from the touch of the earth and we no longer sleep on the earth.

There's a new wave of consciousness emerging called "earthing" or "grounding", which is transforming people all over the world. People walk barefoot outdoors and/or sleep, work, or relax indoors, using energy conductive sheets or mats. New research conducted by universities around the world to investigate the benefits of earthing includes reduced inflammation, less stress, better sleep and more energy during the day. If you are interested to read all about the research about earthing, I highly recommend the Nautilus award-winning book *Earthing: The most important health discovery ever* by Clint Ober, Stephen Sinatra and Martin Zucker. I cannot speak highly enough about this book as it has literally changed my paradigm of health completely.

Earthing is safe for people of all ages. It's not medicine, though, so if you have a medical condition, be sure to consult your healthcare provider. [40]

**Action:** For half an hour every day, connect with the earth barefoot. That's right, just stand on the grass or earth. It is important to note that you should not be wearing any shoes as most of them have rubber soles

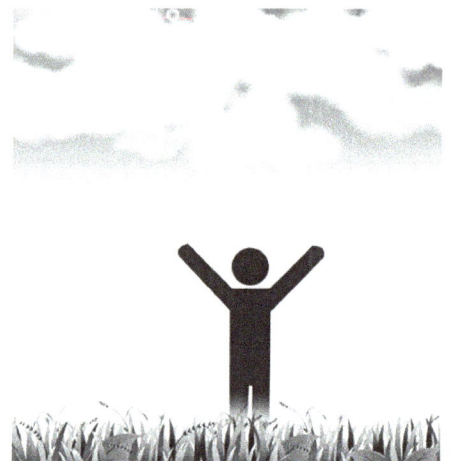

and are an insulator. Therefore, your shoes will stop the flow of free electrons to the body and these a have powerful antioxidant effects. Give it a go for a week and notice any changes to your well-being. My favourite way of grounding myself is to walk barefoot on sandy beaches.

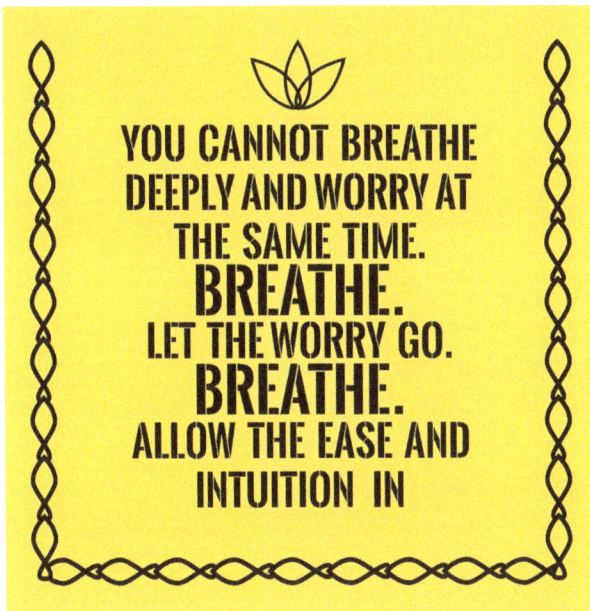

YOU CANNOT BREATHE DEEPLY AND WORRY AT THE SAME TIME. **BREATHE.** LET THE WORRY GO. **BREATHE.** ALLOW THE EASE AND INTUITION IN

## Connection With Air: The Benefits Of Proper Breathing

Most people enjoy breathing fresh air in the morning. We feel good when we have this connection with the air we breathe. Proper breathing is so important as oxygen is an important nutrient for our cells—you might be surprised at just how important it is to your physical well-being and even your psychological well-being. Your breathing can affect your sleep, mood, digestion, heart, nervous system, muscles, brain, and certainly your overall well-being. But by following a few simple principles, you can improve your health, and have less anxiety, less fear, and overall increased well-being.

It all starts with becoming conscious about the way you are breathing. Did you know that we breathe about 20,000 times a day? And that our greatest source of energy is oxygen? The way we can tap into this great source of energy is to return to a more natural pattern of breathing. Newborns breathe correctly naturally, but as we age, we start to breathe more shallowly. By the time we're adults, we're taking 15 to 20 breaths a minute—that's three to four times faster than we should for optimal breathing.

### Harmful Effects of Shallow Breathing

The rapid, shallow breathing that most of us do tells our body that we are stressed so that it begins pumping cortisol, which weakens our immunity. There are many other negative effects. Here are some of them:

- Nervous system: short, shallow breathing results in tension in the body and higher stress levels.
- Constricted airways: shallow breathing makes it harder for the air to find its way to the lungs. We have to work harder and breathe faster to get the same amount of air.
- Constricted blood vessels: shallow breathing constricts the blood vessels, which can lead to high blood pressure, which can make the heart work harder.
- Less overall energy: shallow breathing delivers less oxygen to the cells; the body is in fight or flight mode, which means the oxygen is being used in survival mode instead of for development.

Oxygen is critical to the most important organs in our body. These facts about the brain, heart, and muscles will bring that point home:

- The brain uses 20% of the body's oxygen. A shortage of oxygen causes the brain to work more slowly, and since the brain regulates other bodily functions, they all work more slowly as well.
- The heart beats about 100,000 times every day. A shortage of oxygen to the heart means the heart can't pump as effectively, which leads to bad circulation.
- Shortage of oxygen to the muscles decreases stamina, making the muscles stiff, tense, and less resilient.

### Proper Breathing and How to Do It

Luckily, you can begin to have deeper, more relaxed breathing by following five simple principles.

1. Breathe through your nose: your nose is like a filter that prepares the air as it comes in to be used by the body. When you breathe through your mouth, the air going into your lungs is unfiltered, and that means it's raw, cold, dry and full of viruses and bacteria. Pay attention to whether you're breathing through your nose or your mouth so that you take advantage of the natural filter of your nose. Some people have been breathing through their mouth for so long that they don't know it because the body has adapted to it. But once you become conscious of how you're breathing, it won't take more than a couple of days to begin breathing through your nostrils again.

2. Breathe with your diaphragm: check your breathing for a minute now. It should go all the way down to your belly area for good, deep breathing. When you're breathing with the diaphragm, your chest and belly won't have to work so hard. It relaxes your neck and shoulders, which decreases the pain and the stress, and it helps the lymphatic system get rid of waste products in the bowels.

3. Practise relaxed breathing: it's kind of a vicious circle, but when we're feeling tense or stressed, we tend to breathe more shallowly. This, in turn, makes us feel even more tense. By controlling the way we breathe even in times of stress, our body becomes more relaxed, which leads to better functioning all around.

4. Breathe rhythmically: everything has a natural rhythm from the seasons to the ocean waves, and your body is no different. Optimal, rhythmical breathing helps the body to function at its very best.

5. Breathe silently: coughing and sniffling affect our regular breathing pattern. The same is true of breathing quickly, or even loudly. Oftentimes, we do these things unconsciously, and they can be corrected once we become conscious of them.

Here's what to do:

First, become aware of your breathing. Is it relaxed, rhythmical, silent, and are you breathing deeply through your nose? Second, consciously breathe through your nose. Make sure your mouth is closed, and your nose is not stuffed up. Third, practise inhaling for two to three seconds and exhaling for three to four seconds. Follow this with a pause of two to three seconds. Fourth, be conscious of having a straight posture. This allows you to breathe more deeply and to breathe more easily through your nose. Fifth, be aware of your body in general and how tense or relaxed it is. Make a conscious effort to relax your body. [41]

### Breathing Exercises

Here are two exercises, thanks to Indian mysticism and Oprah Winfrey, that will help you get started on your way to better breathing.[42]

## Diaphragmatic Breathing

Diaphragmatic breathing, improves circulation, eases stress and can speed up recovery from illness. It involves expanding your belly so that your lungs have more room to take in oxygen. Here's how:

1. Lie on your back with your knees bent. Place one hand just below your rib cage and the other on your upper chest.

2. Breathe in slowly through your nose so that your stomach pushes against your lower hand.
3. As you exhale through pursed lips, tighten your abs and let them fall inward.

Do this exercise three times a day for five to ten minutes, then increase that amount. Eventually, you should begin to breathe this way automatically.

## Alternative-Nostril Breathing

This is a yoga technique that should help your relaxation. It reduces blood pressure and can boost your cognitive function. Here's how:

1. With your right thumb, close your right nostril and inhale slowly through your left nostril.
2. Now, close your left nostril with your pinky and ring fingers, release your thumb and exhale slowly through your right nostril.
3. Keep the right nostril open, inhale, then close it; open the left nostril, and exhale slowly through the left. That's one round. Start with three rounds, then add another round each week until you are up to five. Then practise whenever you're feeling stressed.

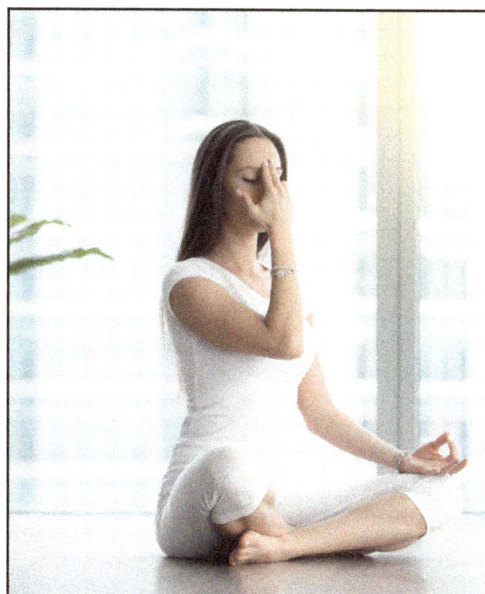

## Connection with water: The Natural Goodness Of Water

If oxygen is essential to life, then so is water. If you have any doubts, listen to these statistics about your body. Your muscles are 75% water. Your blood is 82% water. Your lungs are 90% water. Your brain is 76% water. And even your bones are 25% water.

And guess what? Most of us are dehydrated at least some of the time.

As reported by the London Daily Telegraph, Dr Fereydoon Batmanghelidj, an internationally known researcher and author, has spent his life researching the effects of water on health and how enough water can keep us healthy and pain-free, while dehydration contributes to pain and many degenerative diseases. Here are some of his findings.

1. Water prevents and helps to cure heartburn. Heartburn is a sign of water shortage in the upper part of the gastrointestinal tract. Antacids or other medications don't do anything to correct the dehydration, so the body continues to suffer. The continued lack of water can in time lead to inflammation of the stomach and duodenum as well as other disorders, including cancer in the gastrointestinal tract, liver, and pancreas.
2. Water can prevent and even help to cure arthritis. Arthritis is a signal of water shortage in the joints. Pain medications don't cure the problem and can even make it worse. Drinking water and a small amount of salt is the solution.
3. Water can prevent and even help to cure back pain. Back pain is sometimes caused by water shortage in the spinal column and the discs, which support the weight of the body. Treating back pain with traditional tactics like painkillers, manipulation, acupuncture, and even surgery can eventually lead to osteoporosis and even deformity of the spine.
4. Water can prevent and help to cure angina. Angina or heart pain is a sign of water shortage in the heart and lungs. It can be cured with increased water intake; however, medical supervision is advised.

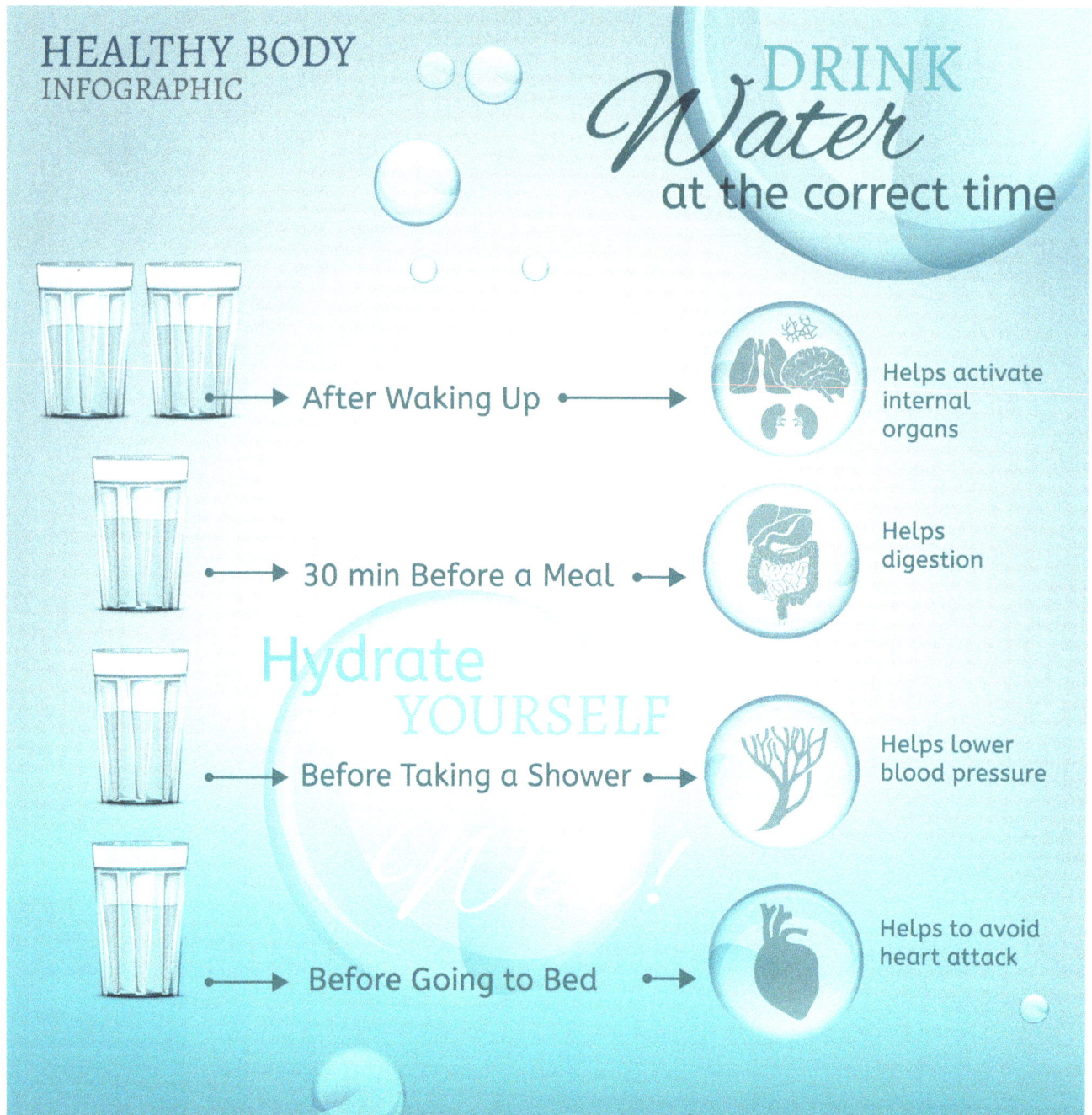

**HEALTHY BODY**
INFOGRAPHIC

DRINK *Water* at the correct time

After Waking Up → Helps activate internal organs

30 min Before a Meal → Helps digestion

Hydrate YOURSELF

Before Taking a Shower → Helps lower blood pressure

Before Going to Bed → Helps to avoid heart attack

5. Water prevents and can even help cure migraines. Migraine headaches are an indication of the shortage of water in the brain and the eyes. Hydration is the solution. Dehydration can eventually cause inflammation at the back of the eye and even result in blindness.

6. Water prevents and can help to cure colitis. Colitis pain indicates water shortage in the large gut. Drinking more water is the solution, but dehydration will cause persistent constipation, which can result in faecal impacting, diverticulitis, haemorrhoids and polyps, and eventually even cancer of the colon and rectum.

7. Water and salt can help to prevent and even cure asthma. The combination of drinking more water and taking more salt breaks the mucus plugs in the lungs, which obstruct the free flow of air in and out of the air sacs.

8. Water prevents and can help to cure high blood pressure. Hypertension or high blood pressure occurs when there is not enough water to fill all the blood vessels that send water into vital cells. The body injects water into tens of trillions of cells all the time. Water and some salt will bring the pressure back to normal. Treating the body with diuretics instead of hydration only makes the problem more acute and in time can cause blockage of the arteries by cholesterol. It can cause heart attacks and strokes. It can cause kidney disease and even brain damage, which can lead to disorders like Alzheimer's.

9. Water can prevent or help to cure early adult-onset diabetes. In adult-onset diabetes, severe hydration of the body occurs with only some cells getting water. Water and some salt can reverse this in its early stages. When the dehydration is not recognised, it can cause massive damage to the blood vessels all through the body. This can result in loss of toes, feet, and legs from gangrene. It can cause eye damage and even blindness.

10. Water lowers cholesterol. High cholesterol indicates dehydration in the body. Water is vital to the proper functioning of cholesterol, which acts as a shield against losing vital water content in the cells. Dr Batmanghelidj advocates water as the free, natural treatment for health and well-being.[43]

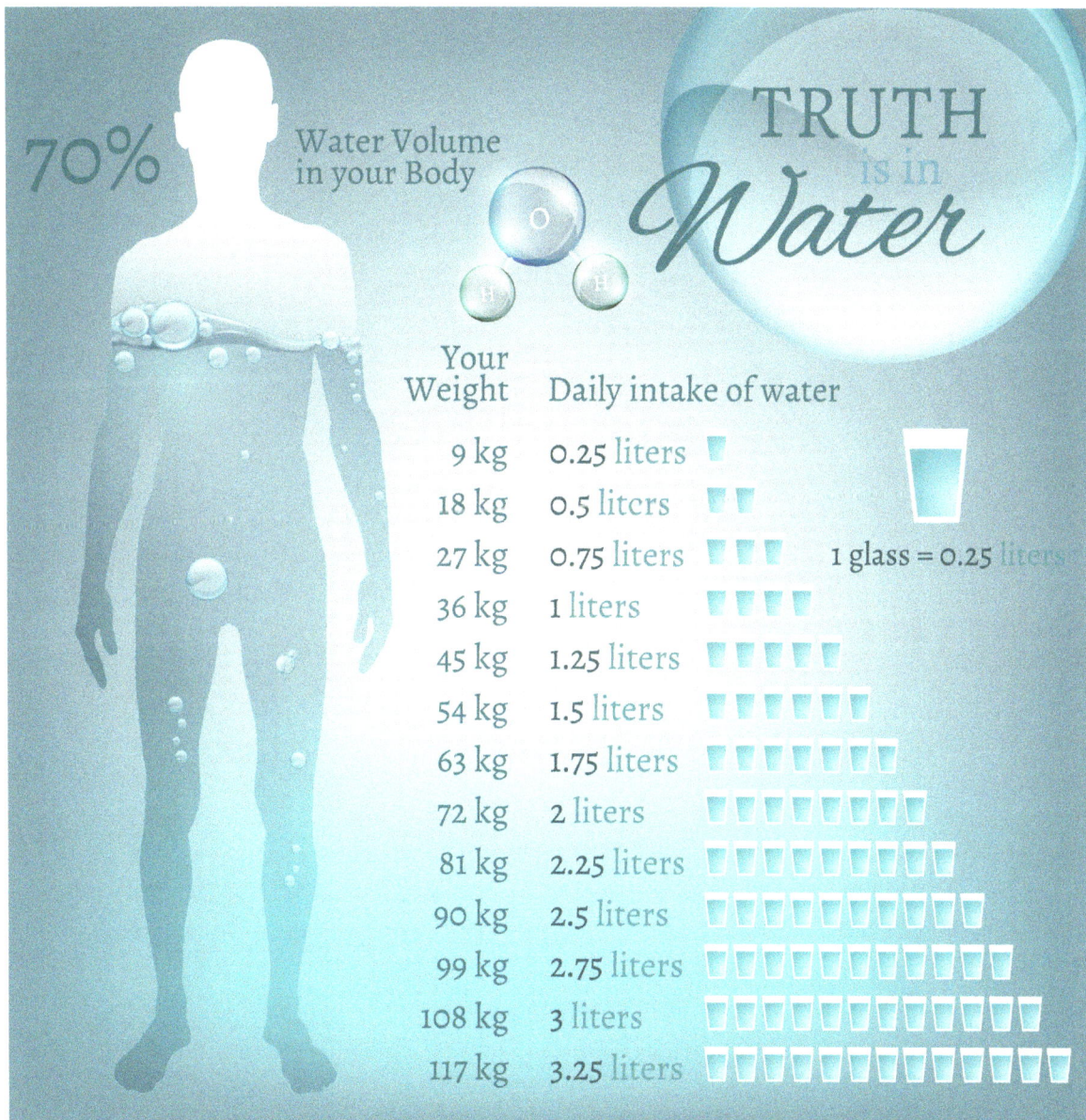

**70%** Water Volume in your Body

TRUTH is in *Water*

| Your Weight | Daily intake of water |
|---|---|
| 9 kg | 0.25 liters |
| 18 kg | 0.5 liters |
| 27 kg | 0.75 liters |
| 36 kg | 1 liters |
| 45 kg | 1.25 liters |
| 54 kg | 1.5 liters |
| 63 kg | 1.75 liters |
| 72 kg | 2 liters |
| 81 kg | 2.25 liters |
| 90 kg | 2.5 liters |
| 99 kg | 2.75 liters |
| 108 kg | 3 liters |
| 117 kg | 3.25 liters |

1 glass = 0.25 liters

How much water you should drink

**Action Step**: Make sure you are always hydrated and drinking at least eight glasses of water a day. It is worthwhile mentioning that alcohol, tea and coffee can make you dehydrated and as a result does not count towards your quota of eight glasses of water a day. How much water are you drinking at the moment? If it is less than eight glasses, increase and take note of any changes in your health.

## Connection with our Surroundings: The Benefits Of Blue And Green Space

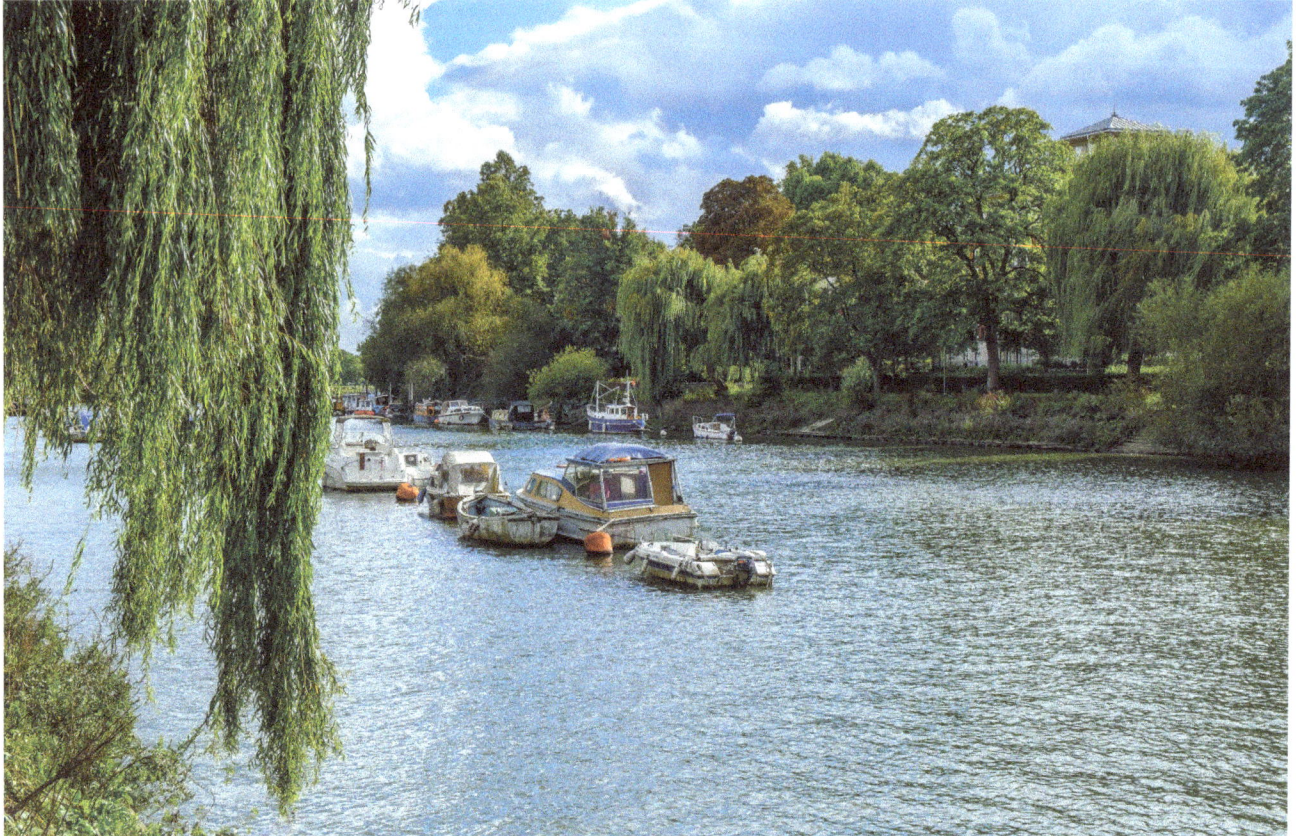

Have you ever thought about the effect of "blue spaces" (seas, rivers, lakes, and even urban water features) and "green spaces" (parks, nature reserves, trails, all open places of natural beauty) on your overall health and well-being? According to recent research done by UK's The Guardian, living with a view of green space is worth up to £300 per person per year in health benefits, and the benefits to residents of living close to rivers, coasts and wetlands are worth £1.3bn per year to residents.

It's been believed for a while now that well-being is related to living near green and blue space, but through recent studies, Dr Matthew White and his colleagues at the European Centre for Environment and Human Health can quantify that benefit. They analysed a sample of 10,000 people over 18 years as they moved closer to or farther away from blue and green spaces. They analysed this in conjunction with other factors such as being married, having a job, and length of commute. The results of the study showing just how important living close to blue and green space was to well-being came as a surprise to even the people conducting the study. [44,45]

Another study performed by Michael Depledge of the European Centre for Environment and Human Health (ECEHH) and Mat White, an environmental psychologist, introduced a variety of images with greenery and water to participants. Their conclusions: "Images with green space received a positive response, but images with both green and blue got the most favourable response of all."

Further studies by the ECEHH and others are using scientific means to tap into the brain to investigate the effect of both green and blue space on stress. One question that is intriguing to all is, "How cost-effective could the benefits of access to green and blue space be in reducing doctor visits?"[46]

**Action step**: Do you have green spaces in your vicinity or park? I have a beautiful park where I live, and a half-an-hour walk there reconnects me with nature. If you want to reconnect with nature, go for a walk in the woods, park or just sit down in front of a river or lake with full awareness of contemplating nature. This will reconnect you to nature and energise you. The most wicked way for me of connecting with nature would be to hug a tree—why not give this a go?

## Connection with the Sun: Sunshine—A Lifesaver

According to Dr Joseph Mercola, over 1 million people die each year due to inadequate exposure to sunlight. Many people avoid sunlight out of fear that it will lead to cancer, but sunlight has life-saving abilities that can actually help prevent cancer. Everyone needs an average of at least 10 to 15 minutes of sunlight every day. [47,48]

A breakthrough study published in 2007 in *Nutrition Reviews* demonstrated how crucial it is to spend 15 minutes in sunlight for your body to produce vitamin D and vitamin D3, which drastically reduce your risk of colon and breast cancer. The researchers from the University of California San Diego estimated that increasing vitamin D3 levels, especially in locations north of the equator, could prevent 250,000 cases of colorectal cancer and 350,000 cases of breast cancer worldwide. Surveys of vitamin D levels from 15 countries were evaluated during the winter when sunlight is at a minimum.

This data was then used to estimate average vitamin D3 among people living in 177 countries throughout the world. It was found that the higher your level of vitamin D was, the lower your risk for colorectal and breast cancer. Even more startling, it was found that in addition to preventing those 600,000 cases of cancer each year, increasing intake of vitamin D3 throughout the world could easily prevent diseases that would otherwise claim close to 1 million lives each year.

It's relatively common for people to believe and even for physicians to recommend that we stay out of the sun to avoid skin cancer, premature ageing of the skin, and cataracts. But the dangers presented by exposure to the sun are much smaller than the benefits.

If you're not used to the sun, it is crucial to build up your tolerance through regular and gradual exposure. It's best to start in spring and early summer to prepare your skin for stronger exposure later. Sunbathing is best in the early morning since there's less chance of burning than later in the day. The healthiest approach is decidedly infrequent, short periods. For Caucasian skin, the benefits can begin within 20 minutes of exposure. It can take three to six times longer for a darkly pigmented skin to achieve the same benefits.

The risk from overexposure to the sun can be significantly minimised by avoiding sunburn, not staying in the sun too long, and eating a healthy diet full of fruits and vegetables. Something that might be news to you is that the antioxidants in fruits and vegetables act to protect you to some extent from sunburn. There is little or no evidence that sun exposure without sunburn increases your risk of melanoma, which is the most severe type of skin cancer. On the contrary, research shows that sun exposure without sunburn decreases your risk of melanoma.

### The Health Benefits of Sunlight

Vitamin D, the sunshine vitamin, influences your entire body, including almost every type of human cell from your brain to your bones. Regular exposure to the ultraviolet rays from the sun that increases your vitamin D levels reduces your risk of all the following diseases:

- 16 types of internal cancers
- Diabetes
- Heart disease
- Hypertension
- Multiple sclerosis
- Osteoporosis
- Psoriasis
- Ricketts
- Schizophrenia
- Tuberculosis
- Myopathy

Even some physicians don't realise that the number one cause of death in Western cultures is not heart disease but cancer, and vitamin D deficiency doubles your risk of cancer. The cancers most strongly linked to insufficient vitamin D are

- Breast cancer
- Colon cancer
- Lung cancer
- Prostate cancer

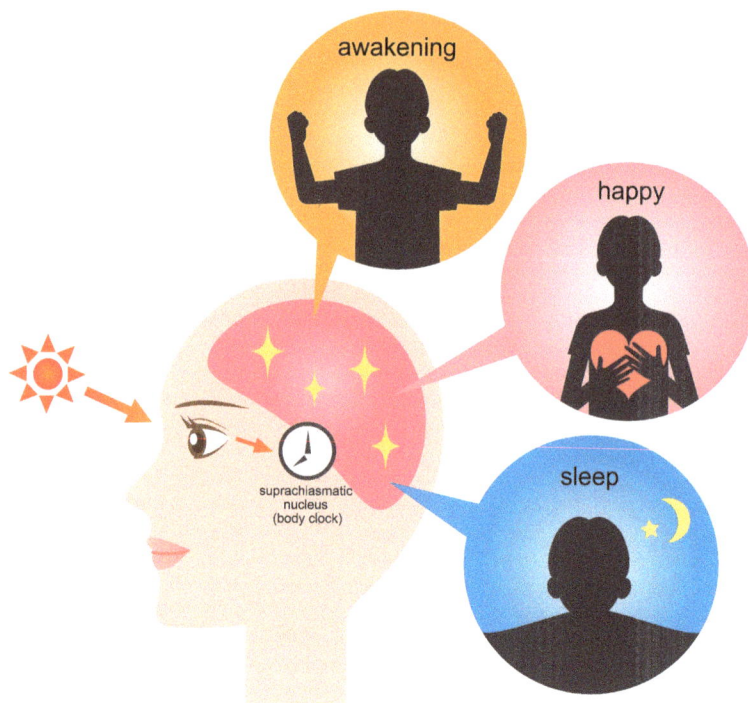

This research was so well accepted that in mid-2007 the Canadian Cancer Society recommended vitamin D for all adults. This is the first time that a major public health organisation endorsed the vitamin as cancer prevention therapy.

Vitamin D is also excellent for your heart. It helps to destroy viruses and bacteria on the cell walls and helps to increase germ-destroying lymphocytes (white blood cells).

Tuberculosis is currently responsible for more deaths worldwide than any other single infectious disease. It spreads through airborne bacteria that enter the lungs and lead to long-term infections. Sunlight has been used to treat tuberculosis since 1903 with so much success that it was adopted by hospitals worldwide. In a study in Indonesia, patients were treated with 10,000 units of vitamin D daily, which resulted in 100% cure rate. [49]

Sunlight has also been shown to be effective against anthrax, cholera, E. coli, this entry, influenza, streptococcus, and other illnesses, while lack of sunshine is the leading cause of maternal and fetal deaths worldwide.

Bear in mind that people respond differently to sunlight depending on age, skin colour, the amount of melanin in your skin, your antioxidant level, you tan level, the latitude, the elevation, cloud cover, pollution, season, time of day, and many other factors. An easy d test will tell you whether your levels of vitamin D are where they should be. It's called 25(OH)D. The optimal level for vitamin D is around 52ng/ml. This corresponds to 4000 IU (international units) of vitamin D per day. An alternative would be 2000 units of vitamin D, along with spending about 12 minutes per day in the sun. If you can, though, it's better to get your vitamin D from sunlight.[50]

**Action**: Remember the sun is not out to get you and give you cancer. Good exposure to the sun is crucial for health. Do not overdo it. The best time to enjoy the sun will be in the morning and the afternoon before sunset.

## PUTTING IDEAS INTO PRACTISE

Connecting with yourself, with others, and with nature becomes real when you take action. These actions can be as simple as smiling at someone or stopping to appreciate a sunset. They can be as varied as giving a friend a ride, finding things around your house to donate to a charity shop, or using the internet to make a donation or to locate a friend you haven't talked to in a while. Whatever connection you make, you will be taking a step to increase your well-being.

Sometime in the near future, create goals for yourself in the following five areas and carry them out:

1. Find a way to encourage or help a friend. Then, if you're feeling bold, acknowledge a stranger—even a smile counts.
2. Do something, however big or small, for your community. Wave to a fireman or policeman. It all counts.
3. Use the internet or social media to do something positive. It could be an email to someone you haven't talked to in a while or looking up some information to help a friend.
4. Find a way, at least for a few minutes, to appreciate and enjoy nature. It's all around us – if you live in a city, there's always the sky.
5. Breathe, really breathe the proper way. You'll feel better.

These are some suggestions. Better yet, find your own ways. You might want to keep a journal of your experiences.

## THE FIVE WAYS TO WELL-BEING APP

Somerset County's Public Health Department in partnership with NEF (the New Economics Foundation) created an app designed to offer guidance and support in learning about and using the Five Ways to Well-being. (The free app can be found in Apple's app store.)

When you sign on, the app will prompt you to use it throughout the week. It tracks your progress and asks you as you go along what is working well for you and what's not.

Here are some examples of what the app's users are doing—maybe they'll inspire you.

- I like to make a chatty comment to the person on the till at the shop.
- I have a chat with neighbours.
- When I'm clearing out old e-mails. I often write an e-mail to someone I haven't heard from for a while.
- I run a craft stall with my Mum and sisters.
- I love chatting with my hairdresser!
- I enjoy the friendship and group identity I get from being a member of a brass band.
- I have a chat in the playground with the other parents when I get the chance.
- I find walking my dog is a good way to connect and keep active. People will often talk to me because I know the dog; it seems to free people up to connect without feeling threatened.
- I am in a book club which doesn't worry too much if you haven't read the book.

- I'm a member of an investment club. The other members are very different people to those I meet today. It gives me a different perspective on the world.
- I meet up with my dog-walking friends in the park for coffee every now and then.

**Action**:

List some of the ways you want to connect with yourself, others, or nature on a daily basis.

# BE ACTIVE

*"An early-morning walk is a blessing for the whole day."*
—Henry David Thoreau

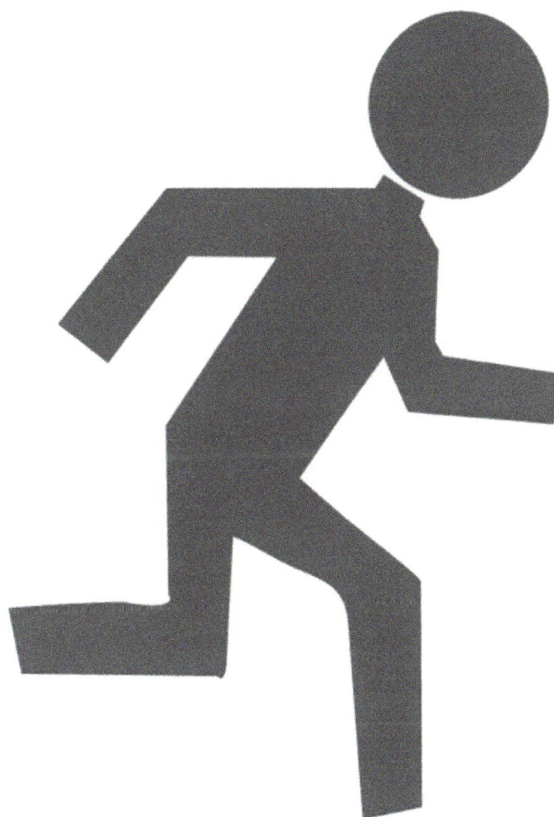

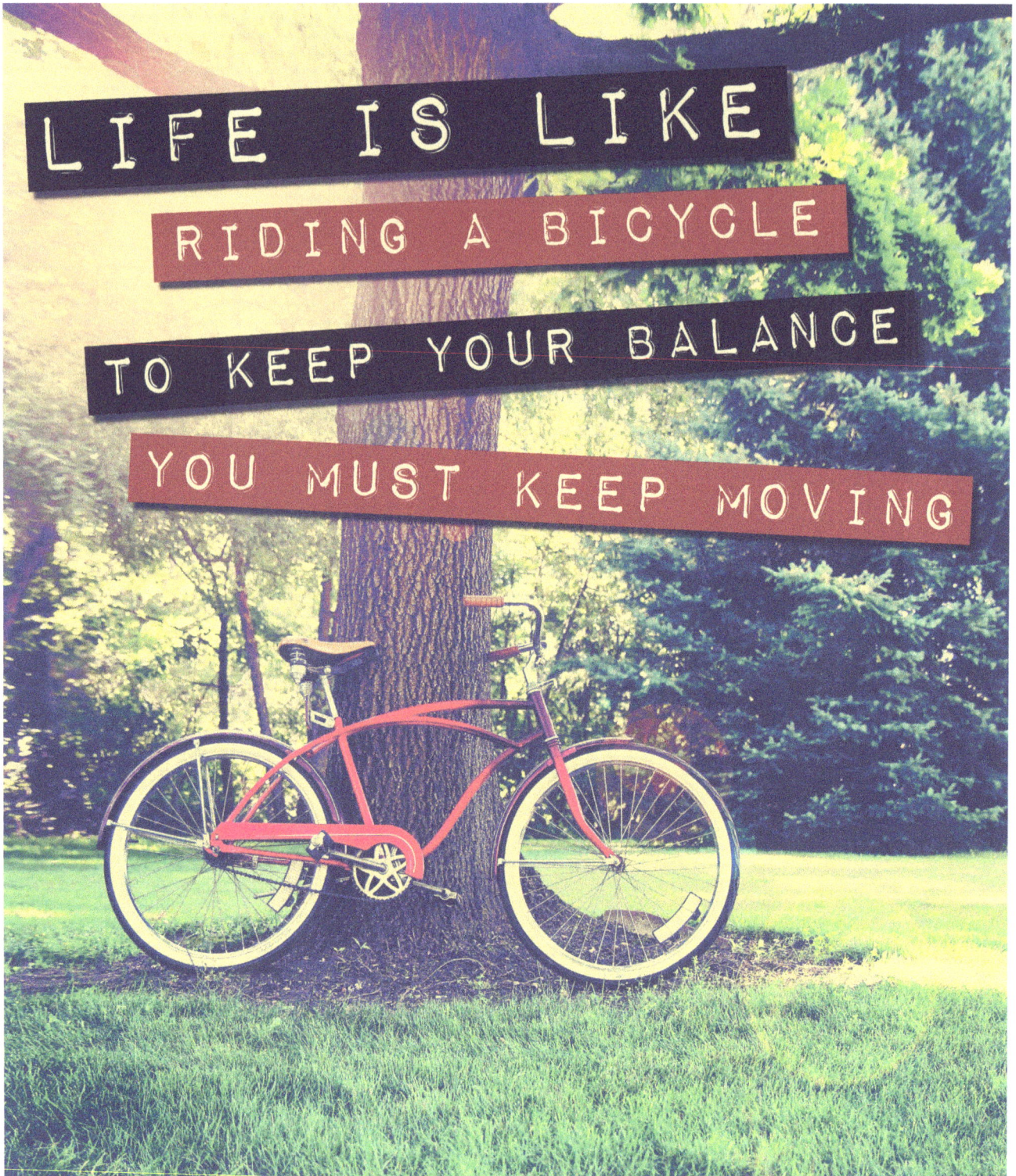

LIFE IS LIKE RIDING A BICYCLE TO KEEP YOUR BALANCE YOU MUST KEEP MOVING

There are no two ways about it. Human beings are designed to move. If we are not moving enough as in today's contemporary society, we have to do some sort of physical activity to enable us to be healthy. Physical activity is a vital part of the Five Ways to Well-being program since well-being includes good physical as well as mental health. It's difficult to experience the feelings of contentment, enjoyment, confidence, and engagement with the world—all the things that define well-being—when you're not feeling well.

Great Britain is at the forefront of raising consciousness about well-being, and this includes taking part in analyses of the effects of physical inactivity on non-communicable diseases and life expectancy.

A July 2012 report in the Lancet indicates a strong connection between the two:

"Strong evidence shows that physical inactivity increases the risk of many adverse health conditions, including major noncommunicable diseases, such as coronary heart disease, type II diabetes, and breast and colon cancers, and shortens life expectancy. Because much of the world's population is inactive, this link presents a major public health issue. We aimed to quantify the effect of physical inactivity on these major noncommunicable diseases by estimating how much disease could be averted if inactive people were to become active and to estimate the gain in life expectancy at the population level." [51]

The study estimated that worldwide physical inactivity causes 6% of coronary heart disease, 7% of type II diabetes, 10% of breast cancer, and 10% of colon cancer. Inactivity causes 9% of premature mortality or more than 5.3 million of the 57 million deaths that occurred worldwide in 2008. So, even a decrease of 10% in inactivity could result in averting 533,000 deaths from disease, while a decrease of 25% in inactivity could avert more than 1.3 million deaths every year. [52]

The interpretation is clear: increased physical activity would improve health worldwide, increase well-being, and reduce health costs monumentally worldwide.

## THE BENEFITS OF EXERCISE

What this means for you personally, just as an example, is that you can decrease your risk of heart disease, stroke, diabetes and cancer by up to 50% and your risk of early death by up to 30%. That's pretty impressive, right? That's just the beginning. You can:

- Lower your risk of osteoarthritis by up to 83%
- Lower your risk of hip fracture by up to 68%.
- Lower your risk of falls (for older adults) by up to 30%.
- Lower your risk of depression by up to 30%.
- Lower your risk of dementia by up to 30%. [53]

Don't we all have at least one family member or friend who suffers from some of these maladies?

What's also impressive is that many forms of exercise are easily accessible to us and completely free. It's a miracle that has been right in front of us all the time.

But wait! Those are just the physical benefits. Evidence proves that increased physical activity can boost your self-esteem, mood, sleep quality and energy, and reduce your risk of stress and Alzheimer's disease. [54]

Here's the problem, though. Almost all of us are less active today than in previous decades. Technology is a blessing but also somewhat of a curse here. We drive cars instead of walking; machines wash our clothes and dishes; we spend our days in front of a computer and our nights in front of a television; most of us have jobs where we don't do any manual work—in fact, most things we do are much easier than they were in the past.

Inactivity is considered a "silent killer," and "sitting is the new smoking." New evidence reveals that being sedentary—sitting or lying down for long periods—is bad for your health. It increases your risk of many major diseases such as heart disease, stroke, diabetes, and leads to weight gain and obesity.[55]

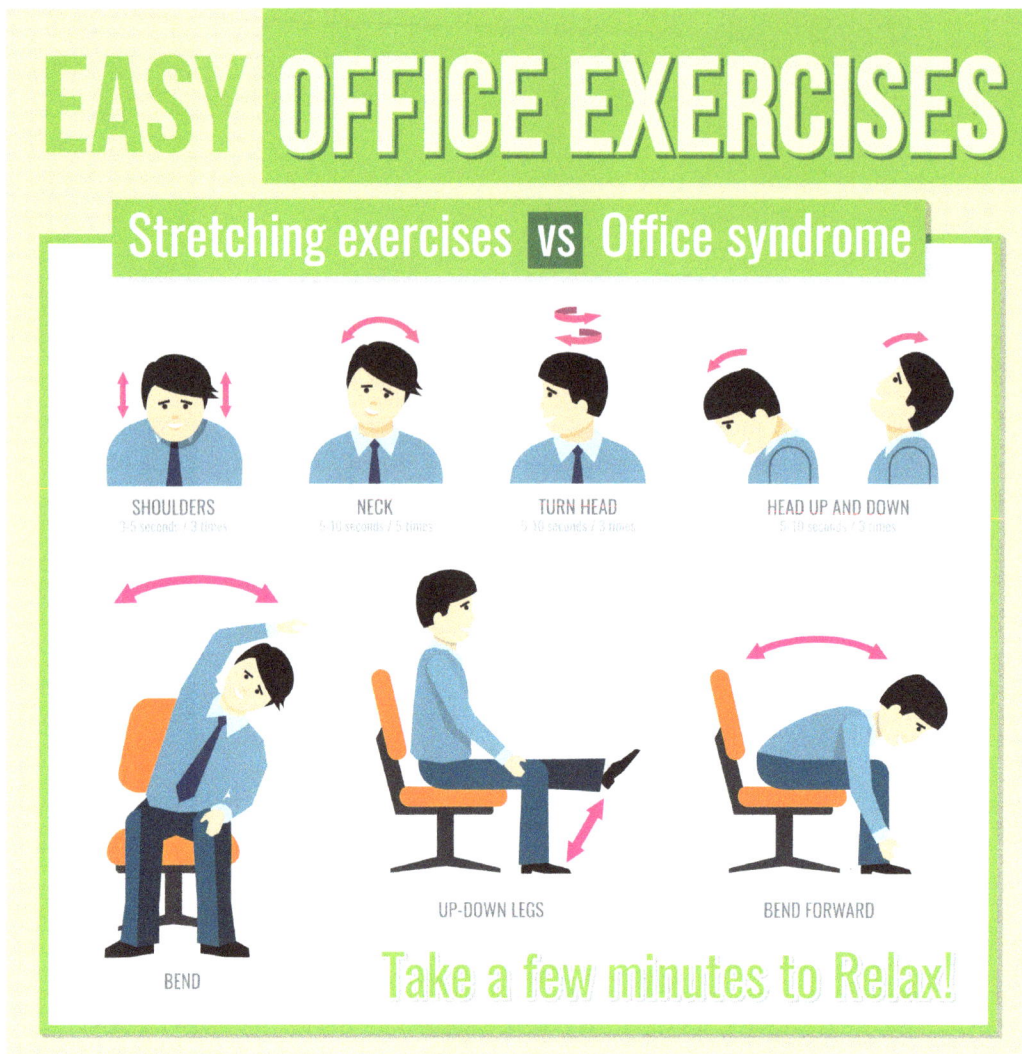

# EASY OFFICE EXERCISES

## Stretching exercises vs Office syndrome

SHOULDERS

NECK

TURN HEAD

HEAD UP AND DOWN

BEND

UP-DOWN LEGS

BEND FORWARD

## Take a few minutes to Relax!

## BEING ACTIVE AND ITS IMPACT ON OVERALL WELL-BEING

In the year 2017 in London, only 34 % of adults walk or cycle for 20 minutes or more. As a result, the Mayor of London wants to address this with his "Health Inequalities Strategy". Many people see the mind, the body and the emotions as all being separate. But what you do with your body actually has a very powerful effect on both your mind and your emotions. Research shows a strong link between physical activity and mental well-being, but this doesn't mean that you need to be a gym rat, sacrificing endless hours there, especially if you don't want to spend your time that way.

The key to sustaining physical activity is to find things that you enjoy doing and ways to fit them into your daily life. It also helps if you share activities with friends and family—this is a good way to motivate each other. It also helps to make a conscious effort to move around if you spend a lot of time sitting each day. For instance, some people do a little cleaning every time the television commercials come on.

No matter what your age or how you spend your time, there are activities that will fit fairly easily into your day. If you're a busy mum, how about

- Walking your children to and from school
- Setting up action activities like swimming with your children

- Exercising during your lunch break if you have access to a gym or pool
- Finding some dance or exercise DVDs you like if you can't leave home
- Finding a neighbour and walking your babies together.

Families have lots of ways to get fit and enjoy being together at the same time. How about:

- Exploring new things to do: a good way to find something you all like.
- Swimming: kids love to play in the water.
- Cycling: go to different places and make it into an adventure every time.
- Asking your kids what they like: working out should be fun for them.
- Getting your children's friends involved: this always makes it more fun.

If you're an office worker, how about:

- Standing and stretching while you're on the phone.
- Walking with a friend during your lunch break.
- Doing a walk and talk, discussing a project while you're walking with someone.
- Getting off the bus one stop early and walking the rest of the way to the office.
- Parking your car farther away from the office building.

If you're an older adult—65 years old or more, how about:

- Finding senior sports or fitness class. You can get fit and make new friends at the same time.
- Doing some heavy gardening. Bending, squatting, carrying, bending, and shovelling are all great forms of exercise.
- Swimming is a great exercise for older adults since it's easy on the joints.
- Joining a conservation group. You'll be getting active, meeting friends, and helping your community at the same time.
- Signing up for a beginners' exercise program in your community. It's a good way to meet people with interests similar to yours.

Becoming more active can be done by integrating small activities into the things you do already, or by consciously choosing to take on new activities that you will enjoy and continue to pursue.

## HOW MUCH ACTIVITY IS ENOUGH?

The Department of Health has formulated guidelines about how much activity we as adults (ages 19 to 64) need to stay healthy. It suggests the following combinations of aerobic and muscle-strengthening activity each week:

- 150 minutes of moderate aerobic activity, such as cycling or fast walking AND muscle-strengthening activities that work legs, hips, back, abdomen, chest, shoulders, and arms two days a week.
- OR 75 minutes of vigorous aerobic activity such as running or tennis AND muscle-strengthening activities that work legs, hips, back, abdomen, chest, shoulders, and arms two days a week.
- OR a mix of moderate and vigorous aerobic activity that equals the above time allotments every week AND two days of muscle-strengthening activities that work legs, hips, back, abdomen, chest, shoulders and arms.

**Moderate Intensity Aerobic Activity**

Any of the following activities are considered moderate-intensity aerobic activity for most people:

- Walking fast.
- Water aerobics.
- Bike-riding on uneven ground.
- Doubles tennis.
- Pushing a lawnmower
- Hiking
- Skateboarding
- Rollerblading
- Volleyball
- Basketball.

Moderate intensity activity raises your heart rate, makes you breathe faster and feel warmer. At this level of activity, you can still talk but can't sing.

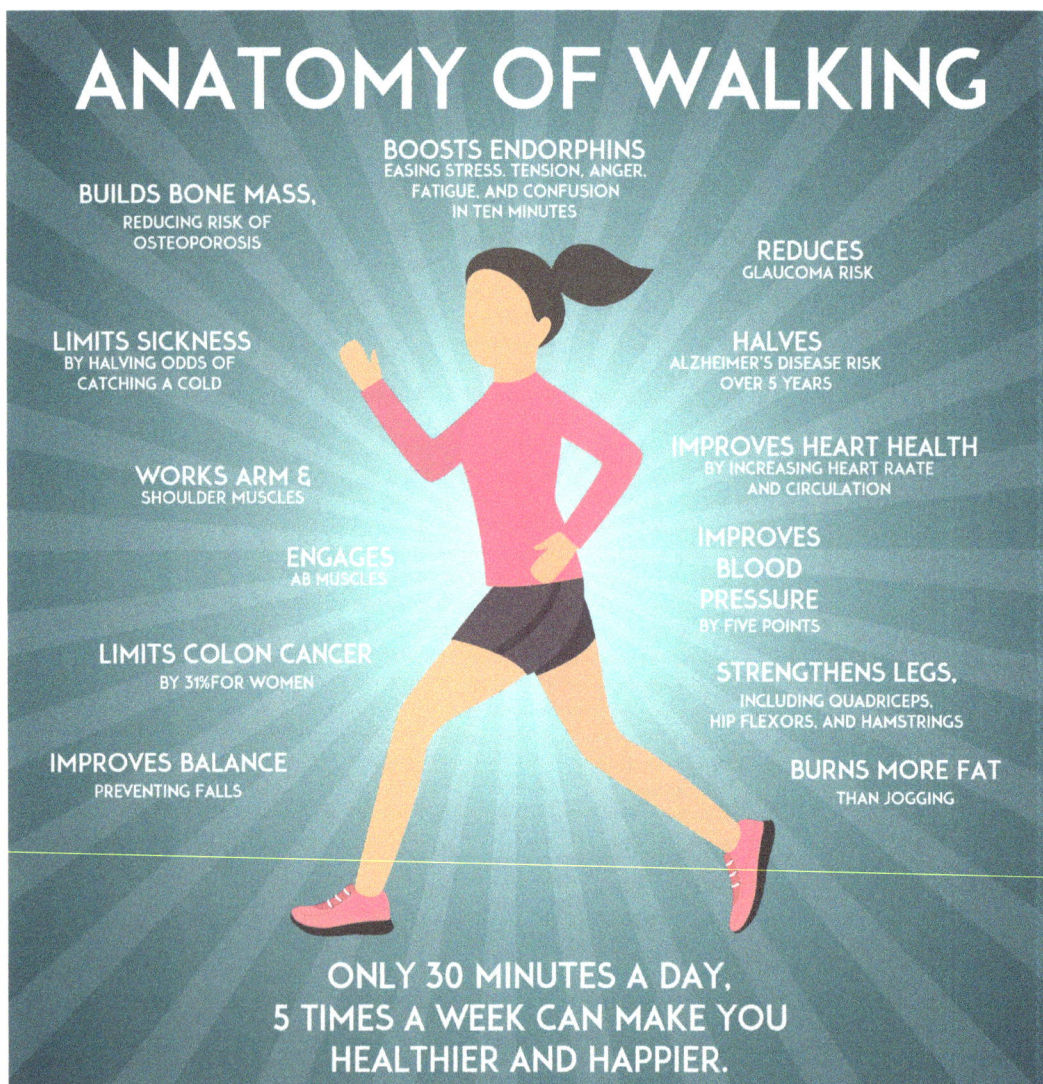

ANATOMY OF WALKING

BOOSTS ENDORPHINS
EASING STRESS, TENSION, ANGER, FATIGUE, AND CONFUSION IN TEN MINUTES

BUILDS BONE MASS,
REDUCING RISK OF OSTEOPOROSIS

REDUCES
GLAUCOMA RISK

LIMITS SICKNESS
BY HALVING ODDS OF CATCHING A COLD

HALVES
ALZHEIMER'S DISEASE RISK OVER 5 YEARS

IMPROVES HEART HEALTH
BY INCREASING HEART RAATE AND CIRCULATION

WORKS ARM &
SHOULDER MUSCLES

ENGAGES
AB MUSCLES

IMPROVES BLOOD PRESSURE
BY FIVE POINTS

LIMITS COLON CANCER
BY 31%FOR WOMEN

STRENGTHENS LEGS,
INCLUDING QUADRICEPS, HIP FLEXORS, AND HAMSTRINGS

IMPROVES BALANCE
PREVENTING FALLS

BURNS MORE FAT
THAN JOGGING

ONLY 30 MINUTES A DAY,
5 TIMES A WEEK CAN MAKE YOU HEALTHIER AND HAPPIER.

**Vigorous Intensity Aerobic Activity**

Examples of vigorous aerobic activity for most people include:

- Jogging or running
- Swimming fast
- Riding a bike fast
- Singles tennis
- Football
- Rugby
- Skipping rope
- Hockey
- Aerobics
- Gymnastics
- Martial arts.

With vigorous aerobic activity, you're breathing hard and fast, and your heart rate has risen quite a bit. You won't be able to speak with ease. In general, 75 minutes of vigorous activity gives the same health benefits as 150 minutes of moderate activity.

**Muscle Strengthening Activity**

Muscle-strengthening activities include:

- Lifting weights
- Working with resistance bands
- Doing exercises with your body weight for resistance (push-ups and sit-ups)
- Heavy gardening such as digging and shovelling
- Yoga.

If you are overweight, you can still improve your health by participating in these physical activities even if they don't cause you to lose weight. Losing weight will probably require doing a more physical activity and/or changing your diet. To be on the safe side if you're overweight, begin gradually and build up to 150 minutes of activity. [56]

## IT'S FREE!

As we said before, one great thing about exercising is that there are so many free choices. Let's start with the ones you can do at home. In only ten minutes, you can get your metabolism revved up and your mood elevated as well. You might be able to find some exercise shows on television, or you could borrow some exercise books or CDs from your local library. Many websites such as
http://www.nhs.uk/Livewell/fitness/Pages/home-cardio-workout.aspx
will walk you through a variety of 10-minute home workouts. You can find

- 6-minute warm-ups
- 10-minute home cardio workout

- 10-minute home toning workout
- 10-minute legs, burns and turns home workout
- 10-minute firm butt workout
- 10-minute abs workout
- 10-minute bingo wings workout.

You will be able to find many other workouts and routines at this website.

## Outdoor Activities

There are many outdoor activities you could engage in either by yourself or with friends.

If you prefer getting your workout outside, walking and cycling are two of the best ways to start. You can go at your own pace, and you can always choose a new location to keep the experience fresh. Walking and cycling help you to stay healthy while enjoying all the green and blue space in your surroundings. To keep it healthy, make your goals about 10,000 steps a day (you could carry a pedometer). Those 10,000 steps will burn up to 400 calories![57]

A brief exploration of the internet will lead you to many, many websites and apps that offer to enhance your walking experience. www.walkengland.org. is one. Here you can find:

- The Walk London Project which details the best walking routes in London.
- The Walk4Life website that provides walking information, routes, tracking abilities, etc. to help everyone enjoy walking more.
- Dr Maps website that shows a series of beautifully illustrated "walking" maps that doctors can prescribe to their patients.
- The Green Exercise Project that aims to demonstrate the value of exercise and walking for mental health. It is funded through the Department of Health. [58]

WalkEngland is one of many websites dedicated to enhancing your walking experience and your well-being. Explore them for a few minutes. You might be delighted!

So simple and so powerful: Walking for Well-being

In a clinical trial, researchers at the University of Vermont in Burlington had 48 participants who were separated doing a moderate activity like brisk walking for 20 minutes or participating in quiet or resting activity for the same time period. The participants were then asked to complete questionnaires at 1, 2, 4, 8, 12 and 24 hours following their designated activity. Researchers found that those who participated in a moderate activity like brisk walking felt a significant improvement in mood up to 12 hours later, compared to the group who were resting. There was no significant difference after 24 hours; thus, leaving them to conclude that regular walking can improve mood and relieve daily stressors.

Another trial conducted at the University of Texas at Austin, participants suffering from major depressive mood disorder were assigned to either participate in an aerobic exercise program or quiet-rest activity. Participants had similar results to the University of Vermont study. Researchers Otto and Smits concluded that "Exercise can be as powerful as antidepressants in treating depression, and, in a more general way, regular exercise is linked with decreased anxiety, stress and hostility."

So, the learning point from those studies is that brisk walking for 20 minutes in the morning can not only uplift your mood immediately but can also uplift your mood throughout the day. Do you want a lifetime of well-being? What are you waiting for? Just walk and be happy! [58b]

# RUNNING FOR WELL-BEING

If you think you might like to begin running, you're not alone, with Gordon Ramsey, Nigella Lawson and Katie Price being three of many celebrities who enjoy it. There are a few guidelines to follow to keep running safe and enjoyable for you as a beginner.

If you're not in shape, you may want to see your GP before you begin a running program. It's best if you begin slowly, maybe start with walking to avoid injury. One thing you do need is a good pair of running shoes so that you can avoid an injury.

It's helpful to keep a journal where you put down the times you're going to run and the routes you will be taking so that it becomes a routine you won't forget. Do yourself a favour and start gently. Warm up before you start each run with some stretching exercises like walking, knee lifts, sidestepping, or climbing stairs. A good approach, in the beginning, is to walk for 30 minutes while incorporating some running from time to time. Then, run for longer intervals until you spend the entire 30 minutes running.

Your posture should be erect with your arms and shoulders relaxed and your elbows bent. Follow each run with a cool down period of walking and some gentle stretching. Consistency is important—it's better to run two times a week every week than six days a week one week and zero days the next week.

With running, as with any exercise program, it's crucial to stay motivated. Here are a few tips to help you do that:

- The NHS offers a series of podcasts with running music and coaching to help you continuously improve your technique, speed and stamina. You can find the podcast at www.NHS.uk/tools/pages/couch-to-5K-plus.aspx.
- Set a realistic goal for yourself. Have a clear, step-by-step plan for what you want to achieve and then follow it.
- Run with a friend. When one of you is feeling negative about running, the other one can offer encouragement. It works.
- Keep a diary or journal. This is where you put your runs, including route, distance, time, weather conditions, and how you felt. This will give you real proof of your progress for times when your enthusiasm is low.
- Keep it fresh. Vary your distances and routes. Looking at the same scenery all the time can get stale.
- Join a club. You'll probably be able to find people at your level, and they'll be a great source of enthusiasm. [59]

**Rebounding**

Have you heard about rebounding? It's really just jumping on a mini-trampoline. It's fun, and it's really popular. NASA thinks it's the best exercise yet! People of all ages can do it while watching television or listening to a CD. The equipment is fairly inexpensive (it varies depending on model—for instance, the Reebok Rounder is about L50). And the benefits are amazing. It:

- Improves circulation
- Increases the capacity of heart and lungs
- Lowers cholesterol levels
- Improves coordination and balance
- Reduces stress and tension

- Improves muscle tone (especially legs, thighs, hips, abdomen and arms)
- Increases energy and vitality
- Boost the lymphatic and immune system
- . . . And it's terrific fun! [60]

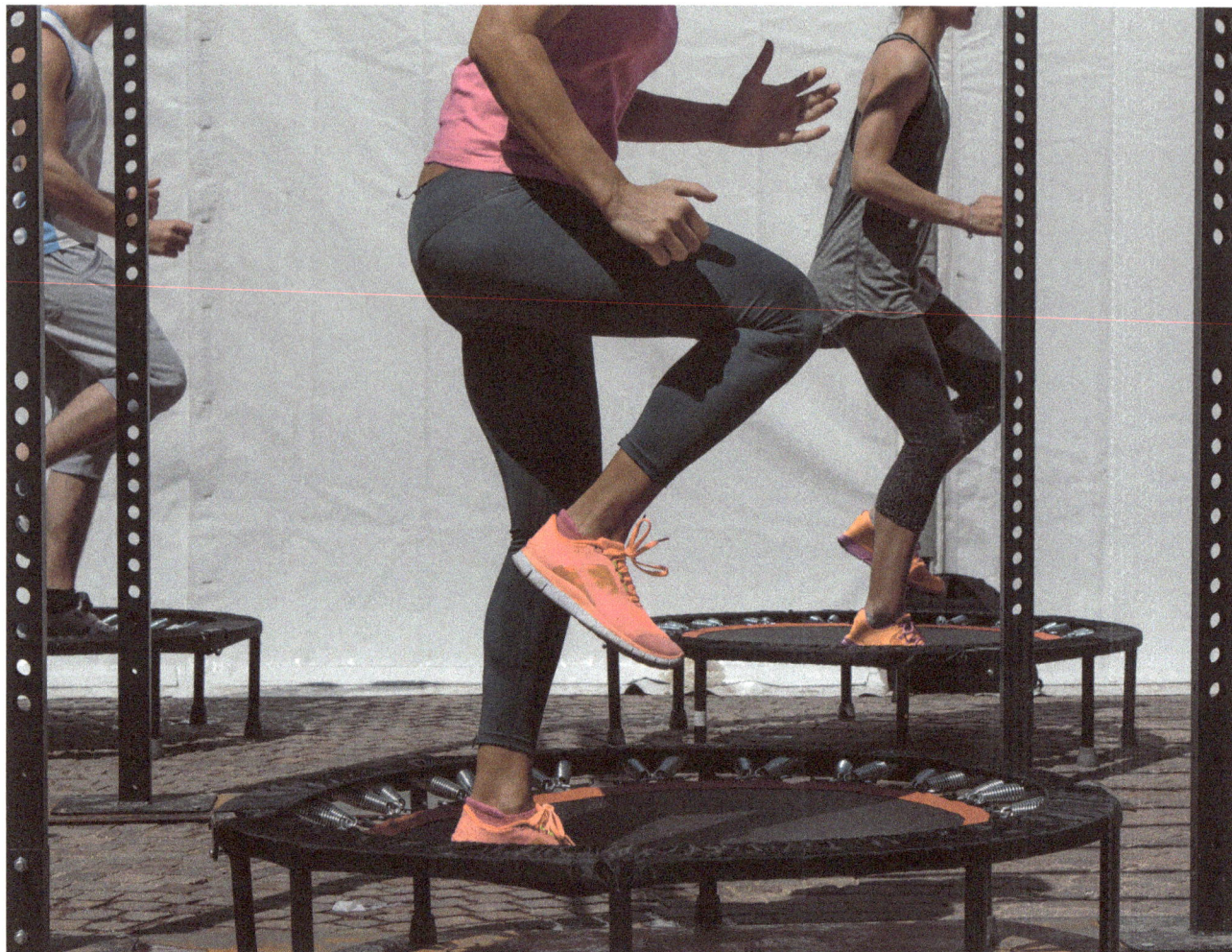

And that's not all. A recent article, The Benefits of Rebound Exercise: 33 Ways the Body Responds, by Dr Walker and Albert E Carter, discusses 33 benefits of rebounding. In addition to the ways mentioned above, we can all reap these benefits from rebounding:

1. Rebounding provides an increased G-Force or gravitational load, which benefits the body by strengthening the musculoskeletal systems.
2. Rebounding protects the joints from chronic fatigue and impact delivered by exercising on hard surfaces.
3. Rebounding helps manage body composition and improves muscle to fat ratio. Rebound exercise benefits you by giving you more control over these.
4. Rebounding benefits lymphatic circulation by stimulating the millions of one-way valves in the lymphatic system. This benefits the body's immune capacity for finding current disease, destroying cancer cells, eliminating antigens in preventing future illness.
5. Rebounding circulates more oxygen to the tissues.

6. Rebounding establishes a better equilibrium between the oxygen required by the tissues and the oxygen made available.
7. Rebounding increases capacity respiration.
8. Rebounding tends to reduce the height to which the arterial pressures rise during exertion.
9. Rebounding lessens the time during which blood pressure remains abnormal after severe activity.
10. Rebounding assists in the rehabilitation of existing heart problems. Rebound exercise also benefits recovery from heart procedures, providing gentle, low-impact circulation.
11. Rebounding increases the functional activity of the red bone marrow in the production of red blood cells.
12. Rebounding gradually improves resting metabolic rate so that more calories are burned for hours after exercise.
13. Rebounding decreases the volume of blood pooling in the veins of the cardiovascular system, preventing chronic oedema.
14. Rebounding encourages collateral circulation by increasing the capillary count in the muscles and decreasing the distance between the capillaries and target cells.
15. Rebounding strengthens the heart and other muscles of the body, so they work more efficiently.
16. Rebounding gradually allows the resting heart to beat less often.
17. Rebounding benefits the alkaline reserve of the body, which may be of significance in an emergency requiring prolonged effort.
18. Rebounding offers relief from neck and back pains, headaches and other pain caused by lack of exercise. Rebound exercise has been shown to benefit body alignment and posture.
19. Rebounding enhances digestion and elimination process.
20. Rebounding allows for deeper and easier relaxation and sleep.
21. Rebounding results in better mental performance, with keener learning processes.
22. Rebounding curtails fatigue and menstrual discomfort for women.
23. Rebounding minimises the number of goals, allergies, digestive disturbances, and abdominal problems.
24. Rebounding tends to slow down atrophy in the ageing process.[61]

And you can have all that while watching television? For some of us, that's irresistible!

## EXERCISE ADVICE FROM EXPERTS

Before you begin your routine, take a minute to look through these general tips about exercising safely and effectively from pros like Robin Gargrave of YMCA-fit, one of the UK's top fitness experts. We've all probably heard lots of myths and incorrect information about the best way to work out. Robin answers several questions that many of us might be unsure of.

1. When should I exercise?
    The time to exercise is a mutual thing, and there's no one right time. Some people prefer the morning, while others have a rough time in the morning. Just don't have a lengthy workout after a heavy meal because you're likely to experience discomfort.

2. Can I have a snack before exercising?
    A small snack is fine but avoid anything with sugar, including soft drinks. Sugar will give you an

energy boost, but it will be followed by a slump. Starchy foods such as brown bread or bananas will keep your energy at a constant level while you exercise.

3. Should I warm-up before exercise?

Warming up is critical before exercising. If you don't, your muscles will be warm, your workout won't be as efficient, and you have a greater risk of injury. Start with slow, gentle movements like walking and gradually build your pace. Take about ten minutes to warm up. This sends oxygen to your muscles, where it works with glucose to produce energy. This way, you'll have better results.

4. What is an aerobic activity?

Aerobic activity is any activity where the body's large muscles move for a continuous period of time. It's excellent for the health of your heart and lungs. It includes running, walking, cycling, and swimming.

5. What's the importance of strength training?

Strength training activities involve short bursts of effort. It burns calories, builds muscles, increases bone density, strengthens joints, and improves balance, stability and posture. Strength training helps you do everyday tasks and makes it easier for you to burn calories.

6. Do I need to stretch?

Stretching is very important. It improves flexibility, balance and posture. Stretch gently, just to the point where you feel resistance. Hold each stretch for 10 to 20 seconds. While you're stretching, breathing deeply and regularly. Do some stretching both before and after exercise.

7. What's the importance of cooling down?

A cooling down period gradually lowers your heart rate while your body is recovering. It can help guard against muscle injury, stiffness and soreness. Cool down by continuing your activity and a lower intensity or by walking and finish by stretching.

8. Should I have a rest day?

With moderate aerobic activity, it's best to do a little every day. With vigorous aerobic activity, such as running, it's good to take a rest day. Over-training can injure anyone, even professional athletes.

9. What should I drink?

It's important to drink fluids while exercising, especially if it lasts more than 30 minutes. Drinking water is fine for a low-intensity exercise of up to 45 or 50 minutes. A sports drink is best for high-intensity exercise and longer exercise periods since the salt in those drinks will help you stay hydrated.

10. How do I stay motivated?

It helps a lot to be doing activities that you really enjoy. Your doctor may tell you that you have to exercise, but you should be the one to decide how you want to exercise. Ask yourself, "What do I like to do?" And do that. Change it up. Set some new challenges for yourself. And keep at it. According to Robin, "It gets easier." [62]

## EXERCISING FOR FUN AND EXCITEMENT!

Walking and biking are great exercises, but they are not the only possibilities. Let's take a walk on the "wild side" and look at a few of the many other exercises you could benefit from.

### Karate

Karate offers multiple benefits from once. It's a total body workout, helping you shed fat, build muscle and improve your concentration. If you decide to sign up for a karate class, check with the English Karate Federation to find instructors with expert training.

### Football

Football is excellent exercise no matter what your level might be. You could even start your own team so that you'll always have a game to go to, you'll spend time with your friends, and the fitness level for all of you will increase.

### Orienteering

If the idea of navigating cross-country with IMAP and the compass appeals to you, you will have a true adventure and exercise your body and your mind with orienteering. Go to www.Britishorienteering.org.uk to find out more about it.

### Climbing

Climbing is not just the mountains anymore. You can do it indoors, too. It builds up your upper body and is also an all-around workout. Surf the Internet to find locations near you that offer indoor climbing and, of course, outdoor climbing as well.

### Paintball

Here's a wild time and a lot of fun for everyone. You're always a part of the action—no standing around with this one. It's a novel way to get some great exercise. Again, find locations near you through the Internet.

### Street Dancing

Why let the people you watch on videos have all the fun? You can join in and get fit while you're doing it. Many organisations offer street dancing classes in many areas around the UK. Go to www.NHS.uk to find out more about it.

### Basketball

Here's a versatile workout that you can play alone, join the team, or create one. It's a lot of fun, and it will get you fit. It's also a great excuse for some time with your friends.

**Ice Hockey**

If you like it rough and tough, this game is guaranteed to get you in shape. It's an intense workout where you burn fat and build muscle. Many skating rinks have several teams, so you're likely to find one at your playing level.

**Skateboarding**

Skateboarding is not for the faint of heart, but it will get you in great shape and get you around at the same time.

**Mountain Biking**

This is strenuous exercise but fun, too. You'll experience the benefits of green space while you're getting fit.

If you go to www.spogo.co.uk, you can find a sports buddy or location for badminton, football, Pilates, skiing, snowboarding, yoga, Zumba, and more. You can learn more about the sport, what equipment you need, how much it costs to participate, and anything you might want to know about sports. It's all there.[63]

## MOTIVATION FOR EXERCISE

Here's where the rubber meets the road. We all know we should exercise; we all know it's good for us. There's no shortage of gyms or trainers or exercise advice. So, why don't we do it? The truth is: some people enjoy exercising, while other people conscientiously stick to a routine because they know it's good for them. Many of the rest of us have a tougher time.

This section contains thoughts and tips about finding the motivation you need to exercise because if you won't do it, knowing how to do it doesn't help at all.

Motivational speakers are fond of telling us that if we want something, we need to claim it as ours, and it will be. Want a good job? OK, declare it, and you'll get it. Well, maybe yes, and maybe no. At first, declarations like these encourage us, and they enthuse and energise us. But studies show that when we don't get the thing we are claiming the first time, we feel bad and don't have the same enthusiasm for declarations after that. Actually, for 87% of us, declarations for self-change give us temporary encouragement but are followed by disappointment when what we want doesn't materialise, which leaves us with a poorer self-image than we had to begin with. [64]

In *The 100 Simple Secrets of Successful People*, Dr David Niven tells us that "Success comes not from self-motivating tricks and declarations of desired outcomes but from a steady, informed effort at progress." He tells the story of David Cynar, who was hit by a car at 15 and was in danger of losing his leg. At first, he became depressed, but David turned inward for hope. He decided that positive thoughts together with positive actions would lead to success. Through rehabilitation, he regained the use of his leg, studied karate, became an athlete and a motivated person in general. Today, David is a successful salesman, a country musician, a black belt in karate, and a volunteer mentor for teens. He sees the accident as the impetus for changing his life for the better. [65]

Bob Harper, trainer and fitness expert on The Biggest Loser, a US television show, provides us with a simple motivational tool that promises more success because it's based on your real opinion about yourself. His plan, "Just One Thing," asks you to find one thing about yourself that you like, admire, or love. It could be your eyes, your smile, or another physical feature. Or it could be more intangible—your sense of humour, your compassion, or another trait. It could also be a skill. What are you good at? Bowling? Baking? We all have something we like about ourselves. Then:

- Name that thing
- Write it down on a piece of paper
- Read it aloud to yourself
- Read it aloud as you smile and look at yourself in a mirror
- Close your eyes and focus on the word and the feeling it gives you.

The point of focusing on one thing about yourself you love is so that you can quickly shift your attention from negative to positive each time a self-critical or self-doubting thought comes to mind. We are all bombarded with negative thoughts, especially if we haven't trained our mind to counteract them, so this "One Thing" mantra will keep you focused on your goals and on feeling positive about yourself. [66]

The second part of maintaining motivation, according to Harper, is to have realistic goals. Be realistic about your strengths and weaknesses and what you like and dislike when it comes to exercise. Choose activities that you like and will more likely continue to do. Then, set up a schedule that is realistic. And if it's a sport you want to improve in—for instance, increasing your running distance or speed— make those goals realistic as well.

The mantra is the seat of your self-confidence, and realistic goals will keep you from feeling overwhelmed. Be realistic about another thing. If you miss a day, give yourself a break. It happens. Move on and get back to it the next day. [67]

Once you start building successes with your workouts and activities, your momentum will probably begin to increase.

One word of caution: Being active is meant to increase your overall well-being. So, choose activities you'll like and want to continue to do. Don't take on activities that are too strenuous for you, and if you need a doctor's approval, be sure to get it. Luckily, we all have lots of options when it comes to getting active. Choose the ones that are right for you.

## PUTTING IDEAS INTO PRACTISE

Do each of these tasks this week or in the very near future.

1. Two can be better than one when it comes to exercising and activities. Find an exercise buddy to go for a walk with at lunch, ride bikes, or take a swim. Time goes by faster when you have someone to talk and laugh with.
2. Sometimes rewards can be the sweetest motivators. Reward yourself for your hard work. Pick a small reward like a lunch out after each activity or one large reward like a spa date each month…or anything else you want. You honoured your commitment to yourself, and you deserve to be rewarded.
3. Create an activity chart for yourself, either with an excel sheet on the computer or in a journal. It doesn't have to be fancy. Just make four columns across the top with the headings DATE, ACTIVITY, DESCRIPTION/REPETITIONS, and TIME SPENT. Then, schedule the activity in advance by filling out the date and activity columns, and fill in the last two columns after you've completed the activity. Set it up for one month at a time and put it somewhere you can see it, like on the refrigerator or on a kitchen counter, someplace you can't ignore it. You're good to go for the month!

4. Set up a journal where you record your thoughts and feelings about your activities. Again, it can be on your computer or with paper and pen, and it doesn't have to be fancy. Just record how being active is making you feel. What benefits are you experiencing? What could you be doing better? Have you started feeling better physically yet? What activities would you like to try next? And so on. Anything you want.

5. Try one new activity in the near future—something you haven't done before. How about a walk-and-talk meeting at work? That is, you have a meeting scheduled with someone, so you go for a walk while you're meeting. It could be interesting, fun, and even stir some creative juices. It could be any activity, as long as it's new to you. It might put some zest in your life.

6. Make use of technology like Fitbit, which is helpful to record your steps and even your sleep.

7. Dr John Buckley at the University of Chester found out that the average person spends around 12 hours sitting. Research shows if you stand for three hours a day for five days, that's around 750 calories burnt. Over the course of a year, it would add up to about 30,000 extra calories, or around 8lb of fat. Something worth doing might be to invest in a standing desk, and that would pay dividends for your well-being. After all, Winston Churchill, Benjamin Franklin and Ernest Hemingway had special standing desks while working. It's not a new concept after all!

Here are some examples from the folks at the Five Ways to Well-being app for inspiration:

**Things I Do To Be Active**

- I park in the furthest corner of the car park which is usually empty, so less stressful park and then in joy the little extra exercise from and to the car.
- I take the stairs at work.
- I go to a salsa class, which is not only exercise but it is one of the most social forms of dance periods. There's always a social dance at the end of the evening.
- I go bowling, walking, gardening and cycling and getting started can be the hardest, but once you start the momentum kicks in. Try one thing at a time.
- I walked the dog.
- I walked to the station to catch a train to work every now and then.
- I tried job of it. Just once a week is better than never!
- I grow veggies, chop wood, run and play hockey in the garden with my son to stay active.

# TAKE NOTICE

*"Look at everything always as though you were seeing it either for the first or last time: This is your time on Earth filled with glory."*
—Betty Smith, *A Tree Grows in Brooklyn*

Take notice (Mindfulness)

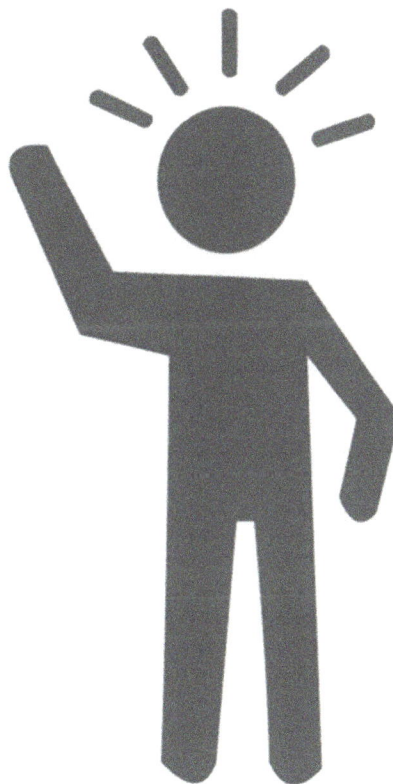

The alchemist was teaching his nephew about life.

"A fight is going on inside me," he told the young boy, "a fight between two wolves.

One is evil, full of anger, sorrow, regret, greed, self-pity and false pride.

The other is good, full of joy, peace, love, humility, kindness and faith."

"This same fight is going on inside of you, grandson…and inside of every other person on the face of this Earth."

The young boy ponders this for a moment and then asked the Alchemist, which wolf will win?"

The alchemist smiled and simply said, "The one you feed."

This is a fantastic story with very deep meaning. As a brilliant metaphor: the two wolves represent to me—mindfulness, (the 'good' wolf) and un-mindfulness (the unconscious mind) or 'ego' as the bad wolf.

Mindfulness, in my experience and observation, brings with it wisdom, compassion, love connectedness and inner peace.

Un-mindfulness, I see in myself and the world at large leads to suffering, anger, greed and destructiveness.

Taking notice (also called *being aware* or *being mindful*) may be the most important part of the Five Ways to Well-being program because it may be the critical key to improving your satisfaction with yourself and your life.

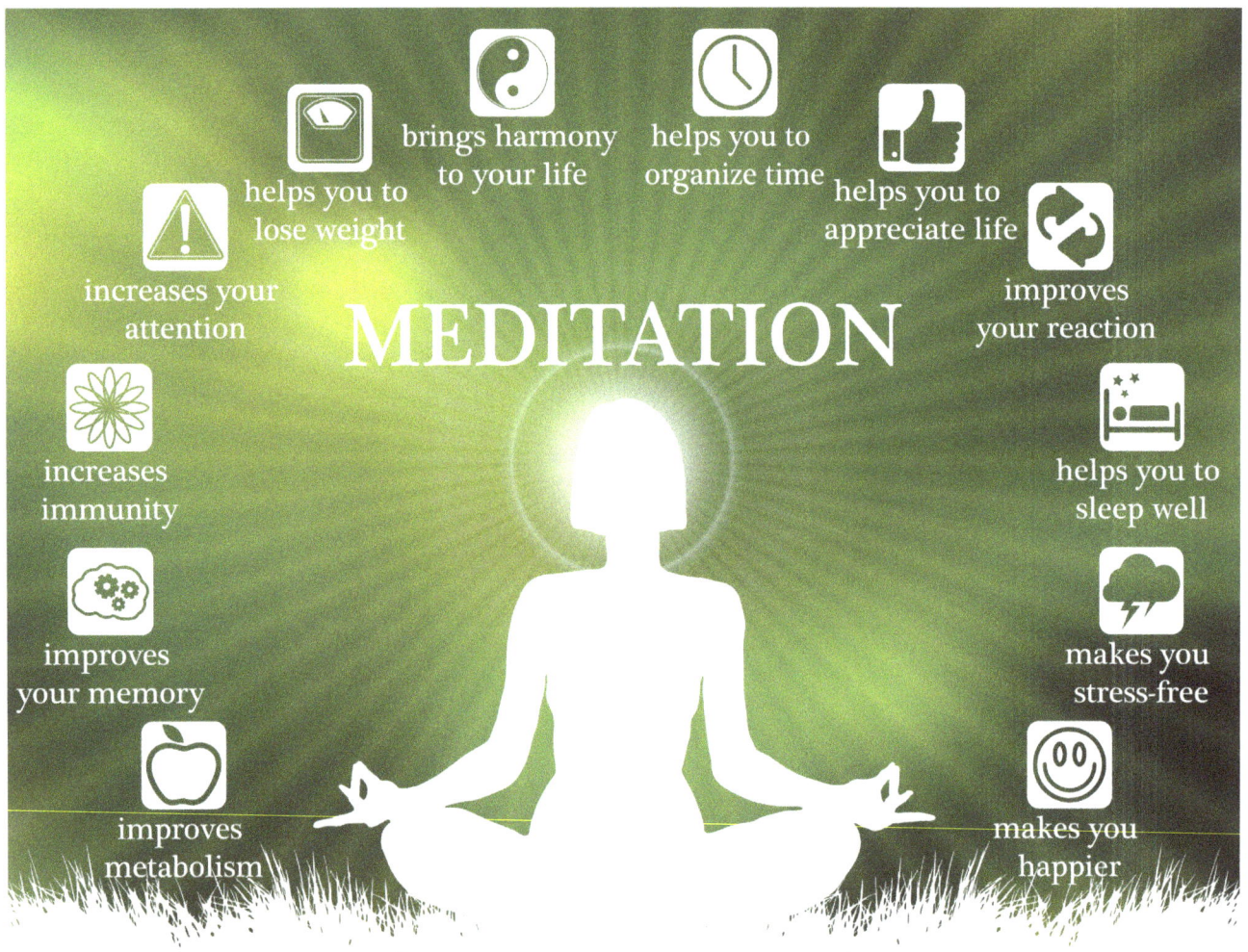

I came across a story the other day about a young man named Barry Ellsworth. Barry might be an extreme example in some ways—but see if you can identify with any of his feelings.

## Barry's Story

Barry and his friends all made six-figure incomes. They financed business deals and made a killing. They drove the most expensive cars, travelled all over the world, dated gorgeous women, wore the finest clothes, and had all the alcohol and cocaine they wanted. But Barry was miserable.

He desperately wanted to know why he was so unhappy. He discussed it with several friends who felt the same way, but he couldn't find any answers that satisfied him. He was bored with himself and his life. How could he find the answers he needed?

Then one night as he paused at a stop light, he had an unusual experience. He saw his own life passing by him on fast-forward as if he were on a movie screen. He'd heard of people having such experiences as they were dying, and he feared that his time might have arrived.

The movie kept playing, so he pulled his car over to the side of the road and continued to watch. He had no idea what was happening. He was afraid and amazed at the same time. Suddenly, he began to hear a voice. He knew the voice was inside his head, but it was so real, it seemed to be speaking to him. This is what it said:

"You just don't get it, do you? Your whole life is a lie. You really think that you are the stories you have made up to impress yourself and everybody else. You have no idea who you are. You think you are your car, your house, your money, your clothes, your drugs, and your women. You think you own them. You believe you are your ideas, your thoughts, your concepts, and your con games. You think you are your illusions. And you don't see that's all they are? Illusions! Stories you tell yourself and others because you have no idea what else to say. Dreams! Nightmares of your own making! And it's all been a lie! Who do you think is watching the movie?"

Then it was over. Barry wondered about what a just taken place. Did he mean that his life had no real meaning? Or had he just missed its meaning? [68]

Barry went on to find the answers he needed. Those answers are very similar to the ones in the Five Ways to Well-being movement.

Do you see any similarities between your life and Barry's? Do you feel that you're doing all the "right things," but you're just not experiencing the sense of satisfaction you felt you would have? Are you working hard and partying hard, but not really enjoying it? Do you feel that there's something missing, but you can't put your finger on what it is?

Believe it or not, that may be the good news. Realising that something is missing is the first step in learning how to be mindful. Mindfulness will fill up the emptiness and help you create a life you can truly enjoy.

## What Is Mindfulness?

It might come as a surprise, but scientific evidence has shown that it's not a great car or a nice house or lots of money that creates well-being. Instead, it's how you think and what you do. It about the choices you make. Professor Mark Williams is a leading authority on mindfulness. He is considered a pioneer in the field of mindfulness research. He's a Professor of Clinical Psychology and A Welcome Principal Research Fellow at the University of Oxford. He is also co-author of the best-selling book, *Mindfulness: A Practical Guide to Finding Peace in a Frantic World*. He explains the science behind mindfulness and how applying it in our everyday lives can lead to greater awareness, productivity and peace for all of us.

Williams defines mindfulness as a way of being, not just a clever idea, but something to practise every day. He claims that there are deep wellsprings of peace and contentment inside all of us—we were born with them—we just have to reconnect with them. In his more than 30 years of studying anxiety, stress and depression, he's found that we try so hard to be happy that we destroy the very peace we've been seeking, but that an authentic, deep-seated love of life is an option for all of us.

His approach to mindfulness is based on mindful-based cognitive therapy (MBCT). It counteracts our natural tendency to solve problems by thinking about them. For instance, when we feel a bit sad, anxious or irritable, our tendency is to try to figure out what the problem is and solve it by thinking our way out of the mood. This actually has the opposite effect. What happens is that our mind automatically starts going through all the previous situations where we felt the same way. Although our goal is to find a solution to the bad mood, memories of similar bad moods only make us feel worse. Our inner critic kicks in, and the problem escalates. We can't find a solution to our mood; we're flooded with bad memories, and we start to believe that we are inept and incompetent. [69]

It's normal to feel some unhappiness or anxiety or stress from time to time—that's just a part of life and one that's bound to come up regularly. But the analytical side of the mind, the side that thinks and judges and plans and delves through past memories searching for solutions, is not our best ally when it comes to handling negative emotions. Here's what happens: you have a problem to solve; your unconscious mind tries to solve it by breaking it down into pieces. Why not? Problem-solving like that is what allows us to finish most tasks and to be productive and successful.

It just doesn't work when it comes to handling feelings. When we can't find a solution through rational, critical thinking, we stall, start to overthink, and begin to brood. We even think that the more we brood or worry, the closer we will be to the solution. But research has shown that the opposite is true. When we start to brood and become moodier, we diminish our ability to solve the problem. Brooding becomes the problem. [70]

On the other hand, the mind is capable of not only thinking but also being aware that it is thinking. This type of awareness transcends thinking. It allows you to step back from the brooding and the negative self-talk you're doing in response to a negative feeling. The ability to do this allows you to see the world or the events in a more objective way. Once you can see past your thoughts, feelings and emotions of the moment, your good mood starts to reappear. [71]

## DOING VERSUS BEING

Williams describes these two types of thinking as *doing* versus *being*. When we're in the *doing* mode, we're caught up in fears about what might happen or regrets about what has happened—we are caught in the past or the future. When we're in the *being* mode or mindful awareness, we pay attention to the present moment and to things as they actually are. [72] This objectivity does two important things: it frees us so that we can actually go about finding a solution to whatever has put us in a bad mood, and it instantaneously improves our mood.

Williams defines the modes *doing* and *being* in terms of seven characteristics:

1.  Automatic pilot versus conscious choice. We all do many things on automatic pilot. In fact, it would be difficult to get through all our routine actions without it. From tying our shoes to doing our laundry to driving, we perform most of the actions involved on automatic pilot. This is a blessing and a curse. It helps us through the mundane things, but we also miss much of our life because of it. Mindfulness brings us back to full conscious awareness, where we make choices and act with intention.
2.  Analysing versus sensing. *Doing* mode thinks, analyses, recalls, plans, and compares. This is truly living in our heads. Mindfulness means getting back to our senses so that we can hear, touch, smell and taste as if we're doing it for the first time. These are simple things that we've learned to take for granted, but when we do them with awareness, we begin to cultivate a more profound understanding of our own inner experience and the outside world. Performing simple things mindfully leads to an increased appreciation for being alive.
3.  Striving versus accepting. Striving means *doing* in a judgmental, competitive way, with toxic tunnel vision toward one goal. Being means suspending judgment and watching the world unfold just as it is

without trying to control it. Mindfulness means you step outside the problem rather than being caught up in it. This liberation ultimately gives you far greater control in finding the most effective solution.

4. See thoughts as solid and real versus treating them as mental events. Sometimes seeing thoughts as solid and real is very helpful. For instance, if you need to get across town in the next hour, you just want to go—you don't want to second-guess yourself. This is true of many, many things we do day to day. But when it comes to feelings, it's helpful to remember that thoughts are just thoughts; they are valuable, but not necessarily reality. They are the way we perceive things in the moment. They can change. This mindful approach frees us from being overwhelmed by a negative thought or feeling. It frees us from wasting a lot of time on negative thoughts that are not reality.

5. Avoidance versus approaching. Avoidance can be a good thing when you know there's a traffic jam you want to avoid, and so on. But a strange quirk of the mind causes us to dwell on things we're trying to avoid. (Remember the old joke about, "try not thinking of the pink elephant?"). For instance, if you're feeling tired and stressed, you could very likely begin to fear exhaustion and burnout by simply trying not to think about them. That's *doing* mode. *Being* mode, on the other hand, invites you to turn toward those feelings that are threatening to engulf you. This will dissipate the power of those negative feelings.

6. Mental time travel versus remaining in the present moment. Research shows that when we're stressed, we tend to think of the past in terms of bad things that have happened, and we tend to think of the future with foreboding. Even worse, we re-live past events and feel the pain again, and we pre-live the future and pre-feel the events negatively. In contrast, mindfulness trains the mind so that you "see" your thoughts as they occur and allows you to live in the present moment. You see memories as memories and thinking about the future as thinking about future. You don't attach negative feelings to either one.

7. Depleting versus nourishing activities. When you're in *doing* mode, you can get caught up in achieving goals to the exclusion of everything else, even your own well-being. This can cause your health, your relationships, and your life to deteriorate. *Being* mode provides balance because you see the big picture more clearly and are more aware of things that are depleting you versus things that are nourishing you. You are better able to deal with things that drain your energy and happiness.[73]

## MINDFULNESS MEDITATION

Mindfulness has two aspects. We've discussed breaking bad "habits" of thinking and behaving that exaggerate our stressful and unhappy moods and deplete our lives. We can break these automatic, unconscious habits by simply acknowledging that they exist and making a choice to think or behave differently.

The other aspect of the mindfulness program is the core mindfulness meditation program. It's a series of simple daily meditations from three to thirty minutes long which can be done anywhere. These meditations are not religious or spiritual in nature. They are exercises that teach you to recognise memories or damaging thoughts as they arise and to see that they are not real in this moment. You learn to observe them, allow them to stay momentarily, and watch them evaporate. You are left with a sense of happiness and peace.[74]

As Williams says, "If *doing* mode is a trap, then *being* mode is freedom. Throughout the ages, people have learned how to cultivate this way of being, and it's possible for any of us to do the same. Mindfulness meditation is the door through which you can enter this *being* mode, and, with a little practise, you can learn to open this door whenever you need to. Mindful awareness, or mindfulness, spontaneously arises out of this *being* mode when we learn to pay attention, on purpose, in the present moment, without judgment, to things as they actually are." [75]

Here's a typical one-minute meditation you might want to try:

1. See direction straight-backed chair. If possible, bring your back a little way from the rear of the chair so that you are self-supporting. Your feet can be flat on the floor. Close your eyes or lower your gaze.
2. Focus your attention on your breath as it flows in and out of your body. Stay in touch with different sensations of each in-breath and each out-breath. Observe the breath without looking for anything special to happen. There is no need to alter your breathing in any way.
3. After a while, your mind may wander. When you notice this, gently bring your attention back to your breath, without giving yourself a hard time. Realising that your mind has wandered in bringing your attention back without criticising yourself is central to the practise of mindfulness meditation.
4. Your mind may eventually become, but it's still on—or it may not. Even if you get a sense of absolute stillness, it may only be fleeting. If you feel angry or exasperated, notice that this may be fleeting too. Whatever happens, allow it to be as it is.
5. After a minute, let your eyes open and take in the room again.[76]

Were you surprised at how simple this exercise is? Here's another one you might like:

## THE HEALTHY CHOCOLATE MEDITATION

Choose some healthy chocolate—either a type that you've never tried before or one that you've not eaten recently. It might be dark and flavoursome, organic or fair trade or whatever you choose. The important thing is to choose a type you wouldn't normally eat or that you consume only rarely. Here you go:

- Open the packet. Inhale aroma. Let it sweep over you.
- Break off a piece and look at it. Really like your eyes drink in what it looks like, examining every nook and cranny.
- Pop in your mouth. See if it's possible to hold on your tongue and let it melt, noticing any tendency to suck it. Chocolate has over 300 different flavours. See if you can sense some of them.
- If you notice your mind wandering while you do this, simply notice where it went, then gently escort it back to the present moment.
- After the chocolate has completely melted, swallow it very slowly and deliberately. Let it trickle down your throat.
- Repeat this with the next piece. [77]

How do you feel? Is it different from the way you normally feel? Did the chocolate taste better than if you'd just eaten it in normal breakneck pace?

In *Mindfulness: An Eight-Week Plan for Finding Peace in a Frantic World*, Professor Williams goes on to present eight weeks of activities devoted to increasing mindfulness. If you're interested, you can find the book on Amazon.

### Benefits Of Mindfulness

Scientific studies in which participants were taught to practise mindfulness resulted in reductions in stress and improvement in mood. As we become more aware of our thoughts and feelings, we can distinguish between healthy and not so healthy thoughts and start to see patterns. We can see when we're getting into automatic thinking and begin to take back our thoughts through deliberate thinking.

Mindfulness or awareness like this let us question whether the thought is helpful to us, and if it isn't, we can change it. This kind of awareness allows us to see signs of stress or anxiety when we begin to feel them, and we can deal with them better.

### Practising Mindfulness

Practising mindfulness means being aware of your thoughts, feelings and body sensations, and of the world around you. You could begin by picking a time during which you made a deliberate decision to pay attention to the sensations in the world around you.

In the same way, make a decision to notice what's happening in your mind. Observe your thoughts as you have them. There's no need to be judgmental; you just need to observe them. As you do this for a while, you realise that they're just thoughts; they don't have control over you. You can ignore them or act on them as you choose. You are in control. With a little practise, you'll get better at deciding which thoughts are helpful and which are just busyness or noise.

You might be interested in pursuing some formal methods of achieving greater awareness or mindfulness other than meditation. You can practise these by yourself or find a group in which you can participate. You should be able to learn more about yoga, Tai Chi, heart math, TrackYourHeart, or other methods through an internet search.

### Yoga

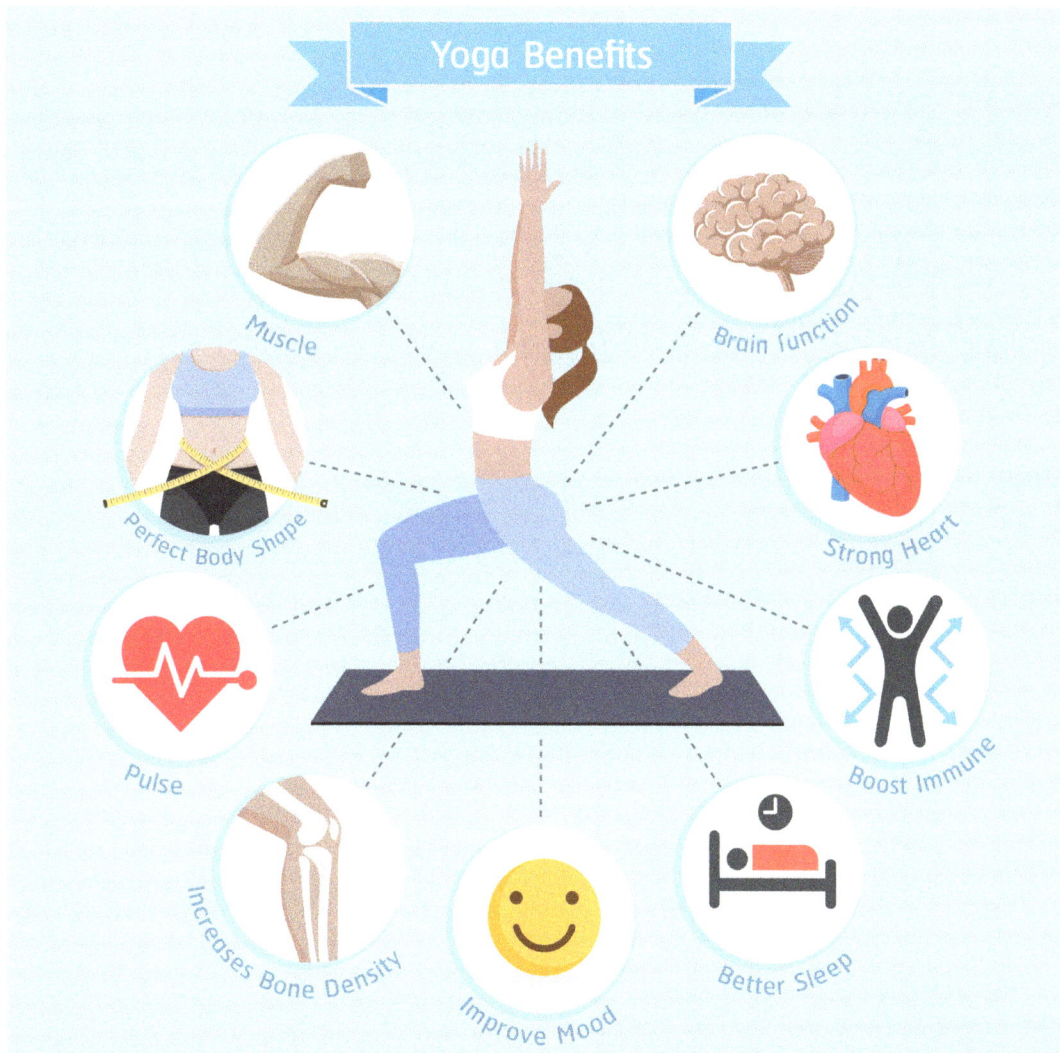

Yoga is a Sanskrit term that literally means union with mind and body. There are various forms of yoga and the most popular one today is called hatha yoga. The practise of hatha yoga originated about 5,000 years ago in India. It concentrates on strength, flexibility, and breathing to increase physical and mental well-being. You will likely be able to find a yoga class in local leisure centres, health clubs, schools, or hospitals.

Studies indicate that yoga is a safe, effective physical activity and possibly assists with high blood pressure, heart disease, body pains, depression and stress. It improves balance by strengthening your lower body, which has the benefit of reducing the risk of falls.

Yoga is a safe activity for people of all ages and fitness levels. You should be able to find a class suitable for you, regardless of your fitness level. There are many styles of yoga (Bikram Ashtanga, and Iyengar, to name three). It's best to choose a class that is appropriate to your level of fitness. Classes can vary in length from 45 minutes to 1 hour and 30 minutes.

You can certainly learn yoga with a DVD but consider trying a class if you are a beginner so that you can be instructed in proper postures and breathing.[78]

## Tai Chi

Tai Chi originated in China during the 1300s and is now practised around the world. It is a soft martial art, designed to work muscles and joints using a gentle and low impact method. It involves positions or postures while standing and taking steps. The legs are used to carry the body, while the arms are moving slowly and gracefully in the air. The posture is continuous to make certain that the body is in unvarying motion. The movement should come from the internal part of the body (the abdomen and the back), and not from the external part (arms and shoulders). It is characterised by graceful, flowing movements.

Tai Chi is good for relaxation and concentration. It can develop strength, balance and flexibility. It decreases stress while boosting stamina and energy. It lubricates the joints and is good for those suffering from arthritis.

There are different styles of Tai Chi such as Yang, Chen and Wu. Some teachers often practise a combination of styles vary in the speed of movement and the way the body holds the postures.

It's a good idea to watch a class or attend a free session before signing up for a course, and of course, if you have a medical condition, consult a GP before taking classes. Since it's a gentle exercise, though, it is suitable for all ages. It can benefit people 65 and over by reducing stress, improving balance and mobility, and increasing muscle strength in the legs. [79]

The practise of Tai Chi and mindfulness has also been shown to improve energy levels, focus and concentration at work. A ten-week evaluation of well-being sessions conducted for health professionals at a community drug and alcohol service in London reports that Tai Chi and mindfulness has significantly had a positive impact on their work with patients.

## Heart Math Technology

For the last twenty years, there has been a steady stream of scientific reports showing the adverse effects of too much stress. Stress accounts for

- A five-fold increased risk of dying from heart-related problems
- Two times the risk of diabetes in men
- A 65% increased risk of dementia
- Two times the risk of obesity
- An increased risk of breast cancer.

The Heartmath Institute has come up with a device, usable anywhere, which monitors your stress levels and helps you reduce your stress at the time of the stressful event. This is important since the negative effects of stress hormones can stay in your body for hours after the event. Also, smooth and orderly heart rhythms are directly responsible for you being able to access higher-thinking centres in your brain. The techniques HeartMath provides allow you to practise mindfulness with results that can be measured. Again and again, participants' physical and emotional states improve through mindful interaction with the HeartMath device.[80]

As a licensed HearthMath coach, I have coached individuals successfully using this technology. I will share one technique called heart-focused breathing that you can practise regularly.

**Action:**

Heart-focused breathing is nothing more than directing your attention to the heart area and breathing a little more deeply than normal. Place your hands over your heart initially, and that will help to direct your awareness to your heart. Imagine you are breathing in and out through your heart. To get good results, Heart Math recommends that you breathe in about five seconds and breathe out five seconds. If I were to prescribe heath math for your well-being and longevity, I would say to practise heart-focused breathing for five minutes three times a day. It is worthwhile mentioning that your breathing should be smooth, unforced and comfortable. With practise, you will gradually establish your own natural rhythm. [80b]

## Track Your Happiness

Studies have shown that our minds wander about half (46.9%) the time. Yes, we spend that much time thinking about something other than what we're doing. Harvard psychologists, Matthew A. Killingsworth and Daniel T. Gilbert, conducted a study using an iPhone app in which they gathered 250,000 data points from 2,250 volunteers. They wanted to understand the subjects' thoughts, feelings, and actions as they lived their daily lives.

They concluded that our minds wander so often that it's pretty much our default mode of operation. (Did you think it was just you? Me, too!) They came to the same conclusions as Professor Williams and the advocates of the well-being movement—a wandering mind is full of thoughts about the past, the future, and things that might never happen at all, and all of it adds up to an unhappy mind.

They measured 22 general activities, such as eating, shopping, walking, and watching television, and concluded that minds wander during every activity except sex. When it comes to happiness, they determined that the actual activity we are doing accounts for only 4.6% of our happiness, while our mind wandering accounts for 10.8%. Finally, they concluded that mind-wandering was the direct cause of the unhappiness. The subjects ranged in age from 18 to 88, with a wide variety of socioeconomic backgrounds and occupations.[81]

This study was the impetus for the creation of www.trackyourhappiness.org, a new scientific research project investigating happiness. If you have an iPhone, you can log into this website and track the factors that are associated with your own personal happiness and contribute to a scientific understanding of happiness at the same time. Here's how it works:

- You answer some questions for statistical purposes. This takes about ten minutes.
- You'll be notified by email or text message and asked how you are feeling and what you are doing. You choose when and how often you want to be notified.
- You receive a report showing how your happiness varies depending on what you are doing, who you are with, where you are, what time of day it is, and several other factors. [82]

This service is free, and it could be fun and enlightening for you, don't you think?

## One More Look At Mindfulness

Are you convinced yet that your physical, emotional, and intellectual health will benefit from you beginning to switch from going about on automatic pilot to taking notice?

Bridget Grenville-Cleave, founding member of the Centre for Applied Positive Psychology and a visiting professor at London Metropolitan University, hopes to convince us. In her book, *Introducing Positive Psychology: A Practical Guide*, she shows us how very easy it is to practise mindfulness. There are five essential steps:

1. Be non-judgmental or impartial
2. Accept things as they are
3. Notice thoughts and emotions as they occur
4. Be fully in the moment
5. Be observant.

Grenville-Cleave lists all the ways that practising mindfulness meditation helps us:

- Better control of emotions
- Decreased rumination (dwelling on negative thoughts)
- Improved working memory
- Better self-awareness
- Improved awareness of thoughts
- Reduced depression and anxiety
- Reduced physical illness
- Decreased emotional reactivity
- More flexible thinking
- Increased positive emotion
- Decreased negative emotion. [83]

She also offers us three choices of ways to be good to ourselves:

1. When you're feeling a bit down and in need of a quick pick-me-up, do one of the following for five minutes: 1. Ring a good friend, one who can be relied on to help you look on the bright side, 2. Go outside for a walk, preferably somewhere green, or 3. Listen to a piece of energising music, anything that will get you tapping your feet or humming along.
2. Create a folder of favourite positive photos on your PC and use them as the screensaver. Every so often when you take a break from your keyboard, a happy image will randomly pop up on the screen and make you smile. Look at the control panel on your PC for instructions. You can also try this on your smartphone.
3. Boost your positive emotions by treating yourself to a special day (out or in), for example a walk in the countryside and a picnic, a visit to an art gallery or a local landmark followed by a nice lunch, a trip to the seaside, a visit to a health spa, a swim, a game of golf or a day devoted to your favourite hobby. Avoid the temptation to spend all day in your PJs, crashed out on the sofa with the remote control, even though this might seem to be the most relaxing way to spend your time. Take your time planning what you're going to do, take your time to enjoy the day and take your time reminiscing about it afterwards.

You can use some of the savouring tips mentioned in Chapter 20. Then try stretching this out into a week of activities. Think of something different to do for 15–30 minutes every day that will boost your positive emotions. Ideas include enjoying a luxury bubble bath or dancing around the living room to some of your favourite songs. [84]

### A Good Time For Self-Compassion

How do you treat yourself? Are you as kind to yourself as you are, say, to your best friend? Or are you your own worst critic? If the answer to that is your own worst critic, you might decide in a hurry that Mindfulness is the last thing you need. A barrage of negative self-talk is bad enough. You don't need to watch yourself saying it!

Well, I certainly understand that. But the problem isn't mindfulness; it's the negativity we're showing toward ourselves. Many of us engage in a lot of automatic self-criticism, often as an incentive to make ourselves do better. However, it doesn't work very well, and it does make us miserable. And the harsh things we say are very likely exaggerations or not true at all.

This is the perfect time to begin acknowledging your self-critical statements as you hear them and realise they're not true and even unfair, and you could even start to replace them with some nice, encouraging thoughts about yourself. It's only fair, and they will go a lot farther to create the overall positive results you desire.

Mindfulness is a powerful tool, perhaps the most powerful tool each one of us possesses. It can change our life from one of chaos where we are not in control to one full of choices which increase our overall happiness. You might want everyone you know to begin to use it, too. That's understandable, but it's also likely that everyone won't see it the way you do. Your responsibility is your own well-being. Insisting that others practise it is counterproductive. Maybe they will come to value it in time.

### Putting Ideas Into Practise

Do these activities this week or in the near future.

1. Create a journal if you haven't done so yet. It can be very simple. All you need is a notebook or a file on your computer. Day by day, write down what you experience as you begin to take notice of the world around you and your own thoughts, emotions, actions, and reactions. No need to judge at all—just record.

2. Choose one of Bridget Grenville-Cleave's three activities listed earlier in this chapter and have fun doing it.

3. Gratitude is a powerful emotion. Write a sincere letter of gratitude to someone who did something good for you but whom you never thanked. Mail it if you wish, or don't. Be mindful of how simply writing the letter affects you for days or even weeks to come.

4. Create a new file on your computer or dedicate a portion of your journal to "Self-Criticism and My Answers to It." When you have a chance during each day or at the end of it, write down the self-critical things you notice yourself saying. Notice the kinds of things you say and your tone of voice. Make up your mind to replace those negative, automatic self-critical thoughts with kinder, more realistic assessments of yourself.

5. Savouring. Just as it sounds, savouring something means being intensely mindful of it in an enjoyable manner. Take a few moments to purposely remember something that happened in the past that gave you great pleasure. Maybe it's going for a swim, maybe it's looking at a sunset, or maybe it's winning

an award. Remember every part of it that you can and enjoy it slowly. Do the same for something you anticipate in the future. This exercise should help you counteract some of your automatic negative memories or negative fears about the future.

## Five Ways to Well-being App

Remember our buddies on the Five Ways to Well-being app? Here's how they are taking notice.

**How I Take Notice . . .**

- I enjoy the smell of newly mown grass when it is there.
- I noticed nice flowers in parks and gardens I pass during the day and take a photo with my phone if it grabs me.
- I like to take time to listen and enjoy the sound of birds singing.
- I take my camera with me when I go out and record the seasons' changes in my town.
- I practise slow breathing exercises a few times a day. They helped give me perspective.
- I noticed the evenings are getting lighter and the seasons changing—little signs that remind me of people in times past.
- I notice how my family are growing up and eating in different ways.
- I reflect a lot on things when I run, appreciate the place I'm running in, feel a connection to the place.

# KEEP LEARNING

*"Live as if you were to die tomorrow. Learn as if you were to live forever."*
—Mahatma Gandhi

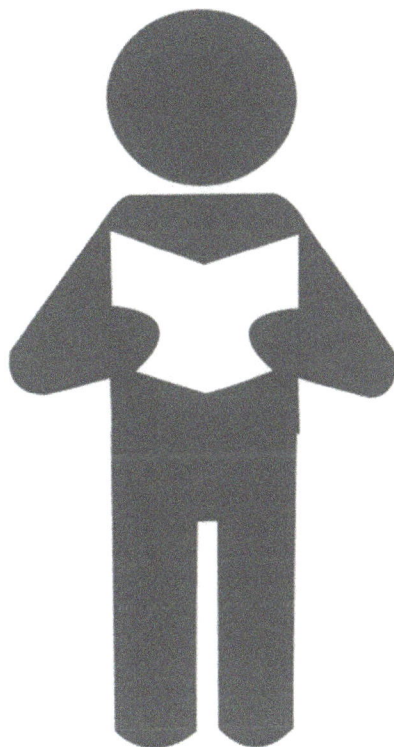

Learning is a never-ending adventure for human beings and contributes to mental well-being. Mental well-being is described as feeling good about ourselves and the world around us and being able to get on with life in the way we want. Studies show that how much we truly enjoy our lives depends on our level of self-confidence, hope and purpose. [85]

Well, that just makes sense, doesn't it? I think we all know that self-confident, hopeful, purposeful people have a better chance of being happy than people who aren't. (Remember, regardless of genetics or life circumstances, we can directly influence up to 40% of our own happiness by what we think and the actions we take.)

But how do we get there? And if we are already somewhat self-confident, hopeful and purposeful, how do we get more of it? That's a great question, and this chapter will answer it.

In short, the attitude of mindfulness (taking notice) is the breakthrough step to well-being, but how effectively we practise mindfulness determines our level of well-being or how much we will enjoy our life. So, we **keep learning.**

This learning is a little different from the learning you did as a child. This time it's all about you understanding on an increasingly deeper level what makes life vital and rewarding in general and especially for you. Each person is unique, so what makes you happy will be different for each person, but—and here's the great news—we all have so many ways to easily explore the things that might lead to greatest well-being for each one of us.

You see, one of the great questions of all time—probably since human beings have existed—is, "What makes me happy?" It's right up there with, "Who am I?" and "Why am I here?"—and the greatest thinkers have tried to answer that question through the ages.

We now have the scientific research that provides proof about what leads to happiness, but all the well-being scientists and researchers I've come across acknowledge that the question has been asked and answered thousands of times. Dr Edward Diener, also known as Dr Happiness, is well known for his research on happiness for the past twenty-five years. He claims that practising "subjective well-being" (SWB) behaviours leads to higher income, better job performance, more creativity and productivity while increasing self-control and creating higher quality social relationships. [86]

As Diener explains in his book, *Happiness: Unlocking the Mysteries of Psychology*, a book he wrote with his son, Robert Biswas-Diener,

"Happiness has been a human concern for the length of our recorded collective memory. Aristotle, perhaps the greatest philosopher of all time, wrote a book on the topic in which he equated happiness with the desirable state that comes with virtuous action and positive life circumstances. In contrast, the hedonists believed that happiness was the result of satisfying passions in pleasurable pursuits. The Greek Stoics, the hedonists' intellectual rivals, believed that it was best to avoid unhappiness through self-control and mastery. In the Christian tradition, Jesus of Nazareth spoke of well-being in his famous Sermon on the Mount in which he suggested that people with good character would be specially blessed."

"European history is packed full of philosophical luminaries, such as St. Augustine and Immanuel Kant, who offered opinions about happiness. In modern times, respected thinkers, such as the Dalai Lama, have turned their attention toward happiness. The Dalai Lama's book *The Art of Happiness* was a worldwide bestseller, proof that this emotion is of mainstream interest and speculation. Although these iconic cultural figures might disagree about the best way to achieve happiness, they all believed that happiness was worth the pursuit. Science offers a new way to examine happiness. Scientific inquiry is not a replacement for religious understanding or philosophical insights, but causality and generalisation add helpful new dimensions to these age-old sources of wisdom." [87]

As Diener suggests, we are in the most fortunate position of being able to take all the wisdom accumulated through the ages and act on it in accordance with what proves to work best, based on scientific evidence in general and for each one of us in particular.

So, your most effective approach to Keep Learning may be to investigate whatever you think might be useful, interesting, and enjoyable to you. Keep what works for you and let the rest go.

I realise that that advice may be a little broad. No worries. We have specific insights and exercises to start you on your way. The best place to start is by getting to know yourself better. The path to your personal well-being must begin with understanding who you are—your values, beliefs, likes and dislikes, strengths and weaknesses, and what really makes you tick. Until you really know those things, you are living someone else's idea of life.

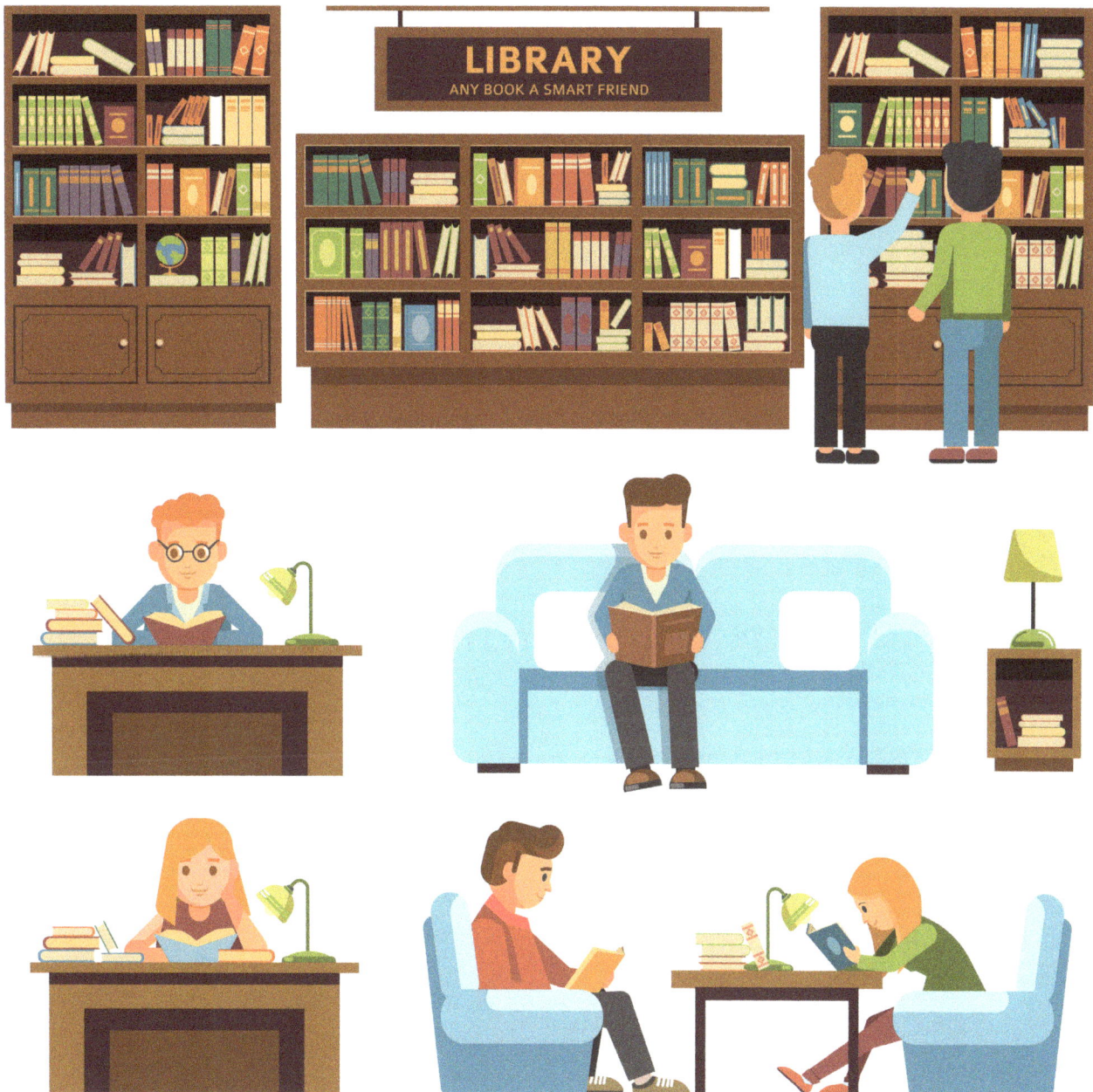

The rest of this chapter is devoted to delving into aspects of you. Be as honest as possible in your answers. We all, every human being alive, have strengths and weaknesses and things we like and don't like about ourselves. Every one of us has fears and obstacles to overcome. Coming face to face with all of it is the first step toward growth. You can't improve something until you acknowledge that it exists. But the results are worth the effort. I promise. It's all about your well-being.

## WHO ARE YOU?

We can learn from philosophy, religion, psychology, the Internet, and even our friends and family, but the place we have to go to find out what we are really about is our own mind and heart. That's the only place where we get the true answers, but it's often the last place we look.

Sometimes, we avoid investigating what we ourselves truly want and need out of a sense of obligation to others. We think that we have to deny ourselves in order to make other people happy, but the fact is that the happier we ourselves are, the better able we are to meet other people's needs.

### What's Your Truth?

Now you know how to practise mindfulness and how to take a step back and watch what's going on in your own life. As you're watching, the more honest you can be about who you are and where you stand right now, the better able you will be to increase your well-being. Remember, "You can't change what you don't confront." In fact, the opposite is true: hiding things from yourself creates a weight that carries an emotional cost to you. But once you let your barriers down, you begin a journey toward openness and emotional freedom.

Have you ever heard the old adage, "Be yourself; everyone else is already taken." That's pretty funny, but it's also true. To achieve the life you want, you pay the price of being honest with yourself about your thoughts and feelings. Keep in mind that there's no right or wrong here—it's your story of who you are. Everything that has happened to you up to this point contributes to who you are. The bad things that have happened are lessons you can learn from. They are not incidents to judge yourself harshly about; they are teachers to show you how to improve in the future.

Life is full of difficulties; it's unfair and even tragic at times for almost all of us. The people are capable of getting beyond those things. Have you ever known someone who seems to have every advantage, but still seems to be living an unhappy, unfulfilling life? On the other hand, can you think of someone who's overcome many difficulties to go on to live a happy, fulfilled life? Probably. History and the news are filled with both types, which tells us that it's not what happens to us that matters, but how we perceive it and how we handle it.

### Understanding Your Feelings

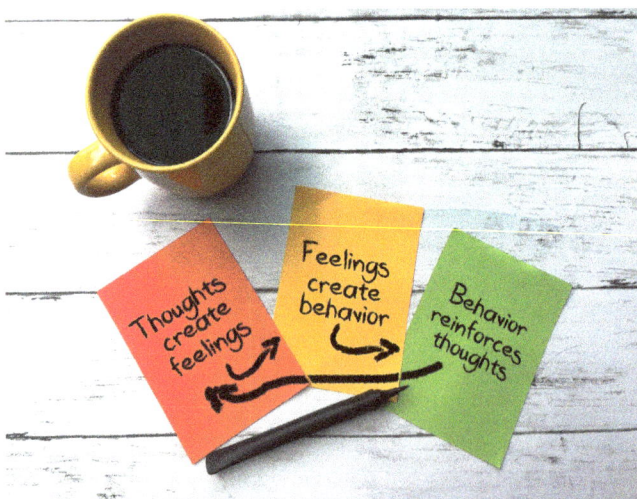

Remember that you control 40% of your own happiness? You do that by what you think, how you feel about what you think, and then what you choose to do. That means that your feelings or emotions are very powerful. So, your emotions can improve your life or diminish it, depending on how you handle them. Now, you can ignore your feelings, you can stuff them down, and you can even tell yourself that they don't exist, but it doesn't really work that way. They're still your authentic feelings—whether anyone else sees them or not—and they determine your happiness.

There are two basic feelings: pain and pleasure. Pain about something in the future is anxiety; pain about something in the past is regret or anger. When you don't recognise these feelings, they can become larger. Anxiety about things in the future (most of these things don't ever happen) exhausts you and can keep you from achieving your goals. If you don't express regret or anger at the time, it becomes distorted. It can exhaust you and even become unmanageable when you express it at a later date.

The best way to handle anger, regret, or anxiety is to recognise it in the moment you're feeling it and deal with it in an appropriate way. This might be a little daunting if you're not used to doing it, but it's a skill you can learn fairly quickly, believe it or not. Soon, you'll be able to express truthfully how you feel about things in a way that others will understand. Then you are being authentic to yourself and connecting truthfully with others. That's a step toward greater well-being all around. Of course, there may be people who won't accept your expression of true emotions, but that is their weakness. They may be able to improve on that with time.

### Are You a Victim or a Victor?

Taking responsibility for your feelings and for where you are in life right now is the first step toward a more fulfilling life. Have you ever heard the expression, "You can be a victim or a victor, but you can't be both?" Blaming other people and seeing yourself as a victim will get you off the hook in your own mind, but it won't get you anything else. You'll never claim the power you need to turn things around. We all make mistakes—some folks think that the only people who don't make mistakes are the ones who aren't doing anything, but making mistakes doesn't make us bad. Sometimes, we are not to blame. Even so, we have to take responsibility, not for what happened, but for whatever needs to be changed. The emphasis is not on excusing the other person; it's on claiming the power you need to change the situation. It's not necessarily easy, but it definitely pays off.

Look at your life right now. Start to take responsibility for each situation. Be honest and ask yourself whether you:

- Are putting up with being treated badly
- Are choosing to feel resentment and anger instead of forgiving
- Are unhappy in your career or relationship
- Are making the same mistakes over and over
- Are living a life that doesn't make you happy
- Are refusing to accept responsibility for who you are and where you are in life.

Rationalisations and justifications are other ways we often avoid responsibility or taking action. Ask yourself if you rationalise or justify yourself in any of these ways:

- Do you rationalise your lack of engagement in life or your lack of progress?
- What reasons do you give for not living as you really want to?
- What do you tell yourself when you don't take responsibility for things?
- Do you say, "I can't" when you really simply don't want to?
- Do you think that your personality traits inhibit what you can do?
- Do you believe you cannot change?
- Is what you believe stopping you from being successful?
- Do you assign blame to someone or something for your failures? [88]

If your answer is yes to some or even many of these questions, you have a great deal company—probably the entire human race at one time or another. But you can change all of these behaviours by learning a few skills. And you'll see that's it's not that difficult. The following self-assessment exercises will help.

## LEARNING ABOUT OURSELVES: SELF-ASSESSMENT TESTS

These first questions will expand on some of the ones you answered before. Use your mindfulness training to step back and see yourself objectively and do your best to answer honestly.

1. How and in what areas of your life do you typically settle for less?
2. How and in what areas of your life have you typically achieved?
3. Do you regularly review your life and reflect on what and how you are doing?
4. Do you think about what in your life is working and what is not?
5. Do you think about what you want to do differently?
6. Do you consider specific changes you want to make in your life and how you will go about making them?
7. Did you review your decisions and consider alternatives before acting?
8. Do you break up your goals into specific, necessary steps? [89]

Dr David Viscott, a well-known psychiatrist and prolific author, says this about the secret of life: "The secret of life is that there is no secret of life. It's all hard work. Yet you still have to find the right work and be free to choose the direction that is best for you. The purpose of life is to discover and develop your gift. The meaning of life comes from sharing your gift with others." [90]

In his book, *Emotionally Free: Letting Go of the Past to Live in the Moment*, Dr Viscott states, "If anyone is going to get in your way to hurt you, it is probably you yourself. Therefore, your weakness admitted is your greatest strength." He tells us that we all have strengths we should build on and weaknesses we should recognise and improve upon. Furthermore, he tells us that, depending on the situation, a character trait that's generally a strong point can become a weak point. And that's true for all of us. The best way to manage our character strengths and weaknesses is to appraise them honestly. When we don't accept our weaknesses, they can limit our strengths. Accepting our weaknesses allows us to become flexible. When we only accept our weaknesses and refuse to take responsibility for our strengths, we also limit our power.

To assist us in analysing our character traits, Dr Viscott gives us a list to examine, which includes the character trait, its understatement, and its overstatement. This list should allow you to examine your own character traits and assess where your strengths and weaknesses fall.

## LEARNING ABOUT OUR CHARACTER: CHARACTER TRAITS ANALYSIS

### Character Traits

| Strength | Understated | Overstated |
|---|---|---|
| | | **Weakness** |
| Believing | Doubtful | Abandons judgment |
| Fair | Unfair | Everyone is so equal no one is treated fairly |
| Forgiving | Vindictive | Doormat |
| Giving | Withholding | Martyr |
| Loyal | Treacherous | Follows blindly |
| Open | Closed | Too revealing |
| Patient | Restless | Apathetic |
| Trusting | Suspicious | Gullible |
| Supportive | Critical | Sycophant |
| Analytical | Guesses | Needs too much information |
| Clear | Confused | Unfocused, sees too much |
| Determined | Disillusioned | Can't let go |
| Frugal | Spendthrift | Self-denying |
| In control | Out of control | Rigidly controlled |
| Intelligent | Plays dumb | Pedantic |
| Wise | Ignorant | Know it all, but no action |
| Measured | Impulsive | Can't risk |
| Systematic | Disorganized | Too many rules |
| Brave | Cowardly | Foolhardy |
| Charming | Irascible | Con artist |
| Creative | Mechanical | Too many ideas |
| Good Salesperson | Skeptic | Easily sold |
| Original | Imitative | Has to reinvent the wheel |
| Poetic | Prosaic | Style over meaning |
| Self-confident | Self-doubting | Pushy |
| Sincere | Phony | Self-righteous |
| Visionary | Nearsighted | Unrealistic dreamer |

The goal is to become your own judge and set your own standards.[91]

## GAINING PERSPECTIVE

Thoughts monitor feelings and behaviour. Your thoughts tell you what to do and many times how to feel. We all have many automatic negative thoughts. Negative automatic thoughts can make you depressed. The more depressed you become, the more negative thoughts you have and the more likely you will be to believe them.

One benefit of mindfulness is that we can recognise negative thought patterns as they arise and then talk back to them or take appropriate action regarding them.

We all experience automatic negative thinking some of the time, and many of us experience it frequently during the day. In A New Beginning: How You Can Change Your Life Through Cognitive Therapy, Dr Gary Emery, a cognitive therapy pioneer, describes some common thinking errors. See which ones are familiar to you. Then take a step back and realise that they're almost always unrealistic.

**Types of Thinking Errors and Examples**

1. Personalising: thinking all situations and events revolve around you. "Everyone was looking at me and wondering why I was there."
2. Magnifying: blowing negative events out of proportion. "This is the worst thing that could happen to me."
3. Minimising: glossing over the saving and positive factors. Overlooking the fact that "nothing really bad happened."
4. Either/or thinking: "Either I'm a loser or a winner." Not taking into account the full continuum.
5. Taking events out of context: after a successful interview, focusing on one or two tough questions. "I blew the interview."
6. Jumping to conclusions: "I have a swollen gland. This must be cancer."
7. Overgeneralising: "I always fail. I fail at everything I've ever tried."
8. Self-blame: "I'm no good." Blaming your total self rather than specific behaviours that can be changed.
9. Magical thinking: "Everything is bad because of my past bad deeds."
10. Mind reading: "Everyone there thought I was fat and ugly."
11. Comparing: comparing yourself to someone else and ignoring all of the basic differences. "Cher has a better figure than mine."
12. Catastrophizing: putting the worst possible construction on events. "I know something terrible happened." [92]

Once you become mindful of your negative thoughts, you can call their bluff with a few very simple techniques: answering, asking questions, and taking action.

*Answering*

Many times, we automatically react to something we perceive as a negative incident by making a mountain out of a molehill. With mindfulness, as soon as we have the thought, we know it's not true or reasonable or fair so that we can answer it right back. For instance, your boyfriend just broke up with you. Your first thought is, "I NEED him." Well, of course you're upset, but do you really NEED him? A good answer would be, "I want him back, but I don't NEED him. I need food, water, and shelter to survive. I don't need a man to survive. Thinking in "needs" makes me vulnerable.

A typical negative automatic statement is "I made a fool out of myself." Well, once again, even at the time you're thinking it, you probably know that isn't strictly true. Your answer to yourself could be, "There's no such thing as a fool. Foolishness is only an abstraction, not something that exists. This mislabeling doesn't do me any good and makes me feel bad." We all have many, many spur of the moment, knee-jerk automatic statements like these. Now, you understand how to handle them.

Once you become mindful of your negative thoughts and answer them back many times, it becomes a healthy habit. In time, you practically stop making them altogether.

*Asking Questions*

Sometimes, our automatic statements aren't so easily answered. Sometimes, we make predictions and then shape reality to make those predictions come true. Dr Gary Emery tells of an instance, for example, where a patient thought he came late to sessions because he didn't like her. He asked her if she could think of any other reason why he might be late. She came up with the right answer—his last session had run over. Sometimes, one good question can turn things around; other times, it might take a few questions.

Here are 20 good questions to ask yourself to combat automatic negative thinking:

1. What's the evidence? Just because something negative happens one time, that doesn't mean it will always happen. It might rain one Saturday, but that doesn't mean it will rain every Saturday.

2. Am I making a mistake in assuming what causes what? The causes for what we are thinking can sometimes be confusing. For example, people often think they're overweight because they have no willpower. But the true answer is a lot more complicated than that. Scientists have determined that overweight is partly biological, social, cultural, psychological, familial, and economic. So, saying overweight is due to lack of willpower is quite an oversimplification.

3. Am I confusing a thought with a fact? Many people tell themselves things as though they are facts and then delete them. Dr Emery gives this example: "how many legs would a dog have if you call the tail a leg? Five? Wrong. Calling a tail a leg doesn't make it so." Question your thoughts; don't accept them as fact.

4. Am I close enough to the situation to really know what's happening? Sometimes our imagination can be our worst enemy, especially when we feel vulnerable or insecure. Have you ever worked with someone who was always afraid he was going to get fired even though there was no reason to think so?

5. Am I thinking in all-or-nothing terms? This is a fairly common tendency, even though most things are on a continuum and not all or nothing. Take a look at the media, for example. We are all exposed to very good-looking people in the media. Some people think, "those people are so beautiful. I'm ugly. I don't matter at all."

6. Am I using ultimatum words in my thinking? Using words like always, never, everyone, no one, is almost always inaccurate and can increase your negativity. For instance, making statements like, "I never get a break" can be depressing and also untrue if you stop and think about them.

7. Am I taking examples out of context? Have you ever just read something wrong? For instance, Dr Emery tells us about a patient of his who was upset because she thought she received a bad letter of recommendation. She thought the reference said that she was "narrow and rigid" when what it actually said was that "She has high principles."

8. Am I being honest with myself? Some of the most damaging lies we tell are the ones we tell ourselves. For instance, "I'll start getting in shape tomorrow" is an excuse that can let you put off exercising for years or even forever. We might mean it when we say it, but we never follow up.

9. What's the source of my information? People tell you things for their own reasons. They might tell you what they believe to be true, but it could be inaccurate. They might not be telling the truth at all. Don't let other people define your reality for you, especially when it makes your reality more negative.

10. Am I confusing a low probability with a high probability? For instance, you're late for work once or twice and say to yourself, "I'm going to get fired." How realistic is that? Counter that by saying, "how often has someone in real life been fired at this company for being late once or twice?"

11. Am I assuming every situation is the same? Do you generalise a negative result in one area to every area? Just because one relationship didn't work out, for instance, do you believe every future relationship will fail?

12. Am I focusing on irrelevant factors? Instead of being defeated by things you can't control, like starving children, wars, poverty, etc., concentrate on improving what you can in your own life and then doing what you can to alleviate others' suffering.

13. Am I overlooking my strengths? Do you tend to dwell on your weaknesses? Instead, think of all the problems you've solved in the past. When you confront the problem, remember those instead of worrying about what you can't do, and then form a plan of action.

14. What do I want? What are your goals? Are they goals that will foster your well-being? If you don't know what you want, it's a cinch you'll get something you don't.

15. How would I look at this if I weren't already in a bad mood? Have you noticed that you can feel completely different about something depending on whether you're in a good mood or bad mood when you're encountering it? It's so true, but take a step back, be mindful, and ask yourself, "How would I feel about this if I were in a better mood to begin with?"

16. What can I do to solve the problem? Thinking thoughts like, "this is so unfair," or" I don't want to do this" doesn't help you to make any progress even though those feelings might be true. Instead, decide on a solution, even if you have to outsource it.

17. Am I asking myself questions that have no answers? This often happens when we don't want to let go of the past. Thinking about ways to change the outcome of things that happened in the past is futile. The past is the past. It's a waste of your energy and your present life to wish for a different outcome. The same is true about unanswerable, negative questions regarding the future that ask "what if something terrible happens?"

    This is futile. Something bad might happen, or it might not. It's irrelevant to the present moment. It's better to do what you can, realistically, and in the present moment.

18. What are the distortions in my thinking? With mindfulness, you can identify the errors in your thinking, and you can correct them. The key is to figure out how you're looking at the situation in the wrong way. Are you overgeneralising? Are you exaggerating? Something else? Pinpoint the error and correct it.

19. What are the advantages and disadvantages of thinking this way? Negative thinking can give you an excuse for not taking action. That can be an advantage if you don't want to take action. But if the best thing for your well-being is to take action, then negative thinking causes you to miss out on improving your life.

20. What difference will this make in a week, a year, or ten years? Are you making too much of the problem or situation? Will anyone remember in ten years that you got a spot on your dress? Or that you made a stupid remark? We all make mistakes and blunders from time to time. It's best to let yourself off the hook and just move on. [93]

### Taking Action

The real point of mindfulness is taking action to increase your well-being. By now, you understand how mindfulness works, you've practised mindfulness meditation, you've stepped back and looked objectively at your thoughts, and you've started challenging any errors in thinking you have. The final step is to take action. Think of something you'd like to do, research it, and do it. How about something new for you and your spouse to enjoy? From a trip to your local library to signing up for a ride in a hot-air balloon, choose something and do it. It doesn't matter if it doesn't work out perfectly. It's your first action, and you have a lifetime of attempts in the future.

Unconscious living means following roles, routines, and rules that give you structure and even security. But it's security with a cost—your authentic, vibrant life. Conscious living or mindfulness means making constant choices. Here's the trade-off: you give up the familiar, even though the familiar might be somewhat pleasant. But here's what you get:

- Expressing your feelings, all of them.
- Admitting the life you tell, especially to yourself.
- Understanding why you tell them.
- Understanding your true needs.
- Letting go, false expectations.
- Accepting yourself as you are.
- Creating your own authentic life—free, productive and happy.

Mindless living leads to frustration and dissatisfaction because you're repeating routines you didn't really choose and that don't represent you. It takes some courage to get beyond your own self-doubt and your self-perceived weaknesses, but once you do it the first time, you'll see that it's not that hard and it's so rewarding.

Making the choice to be mindful is something no one else can do for you, but you can take it one at a time and at your own pace. So, the irony is that stepping up to be mindful may be a little scary initially, but it actually gives you more control than you've ever had before. Take an honest look around, tell the truth and feel your feelings. There you go. It's as simple and as difficult as that.

## The Power Of Change

Have you ever heard the statement, "People don't change"? Do you believe it? Don't we all know people that that statement applies to? Even so, people change all the time. People who want to, that is. It's like the old joke, "How many psychiatrists does it take to change a light bulb? Only one, but the light bulb really has to want to change."

Life is change, and in order to pursue our greatest well-being, each one of us must change. But the truth is that change is scary; it involves risking by stepping on to something new, and so, to some extent, we resist it. What we'd really like is to have the results of change without having to do the actual changing. For instance, you would like a better relationship with another family member, but you dread having to tell that person that you've been wrong some of the time and apologising.

That's just one of hundreds of possible scenarios where the results of changing would probably be great, but taking the initial step is somewhat daunting. So, many times, we remain stuck.

But the ability to change is a skill that we all can learn, and it's one you can strengthen with practise. Inability to change is not a character flaw. It's usually a combination of not believing that you can't change something, not knowing how, and maybe a little stubbornness. In Dr Kenneth Christian's book, *Your Own Worst Enemy*, he gives some great tips about how to practise the skill of changing:

- Change is easier when you focus on one thing at a time.
- Take a long-range perspective to change. You need commitment and persistence to change. You might encounter obstacles and temporary setbacks. Looking at your long-term goal will help you get through these.
- You can't change the past. No amount of change can do that. Fortunately, you don't have to change the past since you can change what happens from this minute on if you decide to.
- You are not the problem. The problem is always what you choose to do. If you have chosen less than successful actions in the past, your mindfulness will allow you to make better choices from now on.

- Change is not something that happens to you; it is something you do. Remember, you want to be a victor, not a victim. You choose the change, and you take action on it.
- Change is a learning process. You won't necessarily get it all right at once. We usually don't.
- Failure is necessary for learning. We all wish that weren't true, but it is. Thomas Edison learned 10,000 lessons before they brought him to invent the light bulb. The same is true for us. Something we tried might have failed, but we ourselves are not failures, and we've come that much closer to succeeding. As has been said before, "The only failure is not trying."[94]

One thing to remember is that the real point of learning is to put it to use in some way in your life. For some people, taking action is hard, so they have a lot of great ideas that they never really benefit from. We have a natural tendency to fear change—even when it's for the better. So, when you need to put something you've learned into action, use mindfulness to realise that this will be for your good, and take action.

## PUTTING IDEAS INTO PRACTISE

Do these exercises this week or in the near future.

1. Each morning and each evening take a few minutes to visualise yourself happily living your best life. What would it be like? Imagine every detail. Set the scene specifically and clearly so that you can feel the experience. What are you wearing? What time of day is it? How do you feel? What else do you notice? What will you do today to increase your well-being?

2. Visualise yourself in five different situations where you are overcoming obstacles. It could be a situation from your past that you wish had ended differently. (It's ok to think about the past in this exercise.) It could be a scene in the present or something that might happen in the future. See yourself as facing the problem and resolving it in a favourable light.

3. Let's work on perception today. Have you ever had a good friend who believes exactly the opposite of what you believe about some things? Interesting, isn't it? If you investigate a little, you might find that your beliefs are based on the different facts you know or choose to believe about the issue. With mindfulness, we can enlist the amazing power of changing our mind when we uncover better information. What's the truth about the following statements? Are they true, false, or does the truth lie somewhere in between and possibly change with the circumstances?

    1. The world is a beautiful place.
    2. No obstacle is too great to overcome.
    3. Life is pain.
    4. Nature is bountiful.
    5. People are basically selfish.
    6. We can save the entire planet if we really want to.
    7. We deserve the best that life has to offer.
    8. Pride goes before a fall.
    9. The grass is always greener on the other side.
    10. All that glitters is not gold.

4. Have you ever heard the expression, "When the student is ready, the teacher appears"? In this exercise, you are the student and life is the teacher. As you go through your day today, ask yourself many times,

"What do I need to learn in this situation?" What is the situation telling you? Just by asking the question, you will probably cause many things to show up. This might be an exercise you want to practise every day.

5.  Decide on some things you want to change in your life. Start with something small and then go on to larger things. Focus on changing one thing at a time. Dr Kenneth Christian describes the process of change in these steps:

    1.  Pre-contemplation: You know something is not right, but you're not quite sure what is wrong. If you ignore your discomfort or find sufficient distractions, you can stay in this stage indefinitely.
    2.  Contemplation: At this stage, you know there's a problem and begin to discuss with yourself the ways you might go about changing it. You're not yet committed to the change.
    3.  Preparation: Now the change is becoming real as you make a step-by-step plan. You're doing the research you need to do and putting things in place to take action. You are also getting accustomed to the idea of the change. You set the date to begin.
    4.  Action: Now you're taking the actions you planned, and the change starts to be obvious to others.
    5.  Maintenance: This is a vital phase. Your actions are in place, but you need to maintain them so that you don't go back to your old ways. Nurture, solidify, and strengthen your new habit. Recognise that your new habit is improving your life. [95]

Here's what our friends at the Five Ways to Well-being app are doing to keep learning:

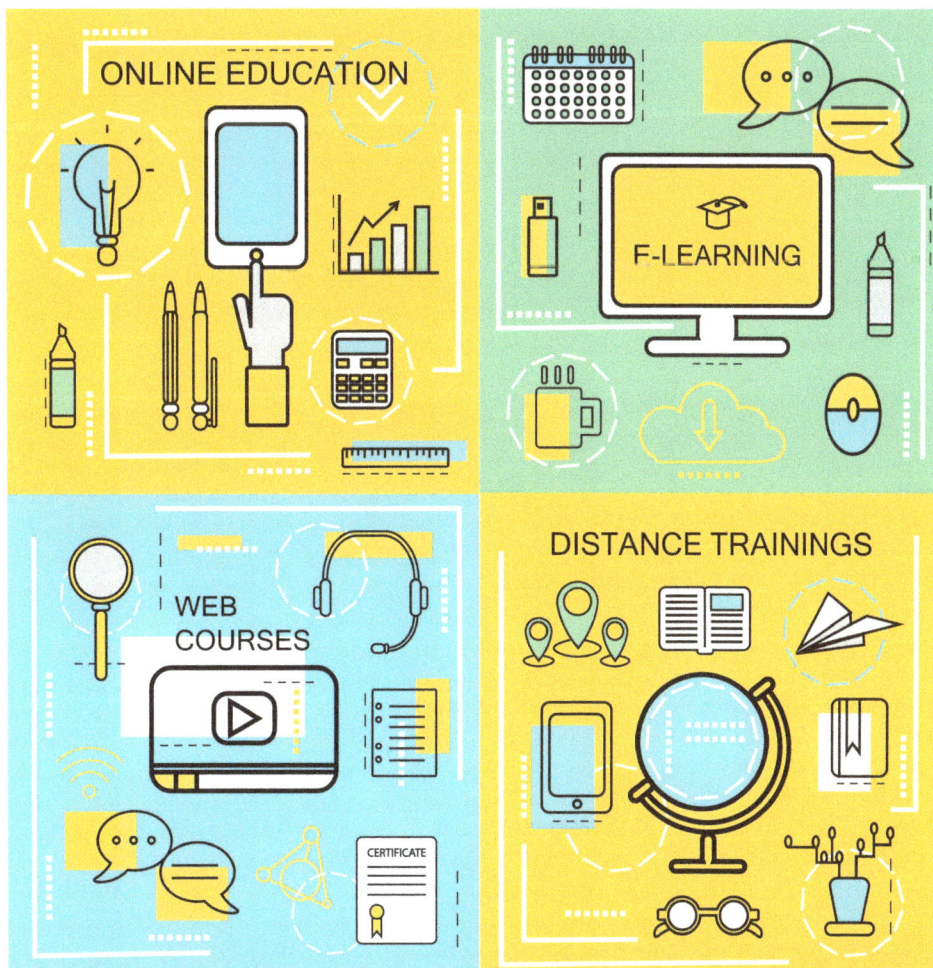

## WAYS I KEEP LEARNING . . .

- I listen to BBC Radio 4 in the car and enjoy all the new and interesting facts I learn.
- I go to community education classes to learn a new language: today, to sew and to do basic car maintenance. It all lets me learn things one small part at the time.
- I've started learning to play an instrument and joined a training band. It's helped me connect too.
- I keep my mind open and prepared to do things differently where possible.
- I change routines and acknowledge the wisdom that comes with experience.

"Research highlights that learning on an ongoing basis builds the key determinants of health and wellbeing including literacy, skills, awareness and empathy" The Reading Agency

# GIVE

*"It's not how much we give but how much love we put into giving."*
—Mother Teresa

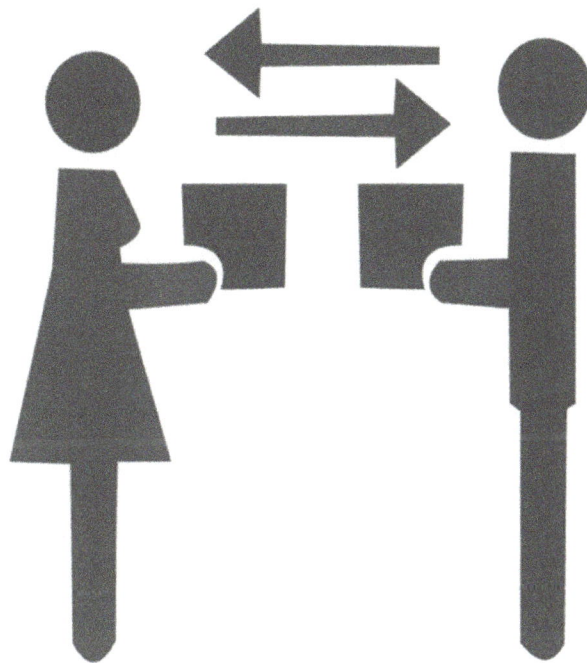

I have organised a number of health and well-being events in London, and I have donated thousands of pounds to charity over the years. Funnily enough, when I have started to do it, I was doing it to help to make a difference to my community, to other people's lives and to make the world we are living a better place. Little did I know that doing charity work would impact on my well-being in a positive way. Indeed, it has! And this chapter highlights the research about giving. It is common knowledge that giving is a good thing we do for other people. But this is a book about YOUR well-being, so this is a chapter about how giving (and receiving) will help you. Many of us think that we "should" give, but we put it off until it's more convenient. Receiving is uncomfortable for many of us because we feel it's somehow selfish and we're afraid it obligates us to reciprocate. Giving and receiving are actually two sides of the same coin. They can both lead you to cultivate an open heart—a sure path to your greater well-being.

In fact, we cannot be compassionate to our fellow human being if we are not living in the moment. Andy Bradley, who researches and has been running compassionate circles in the UK for years, found that being able to give and receive genuine compliments with undivided attention bridges the lost soul of the human being and this can be very healing.

## AN OPEN HEART

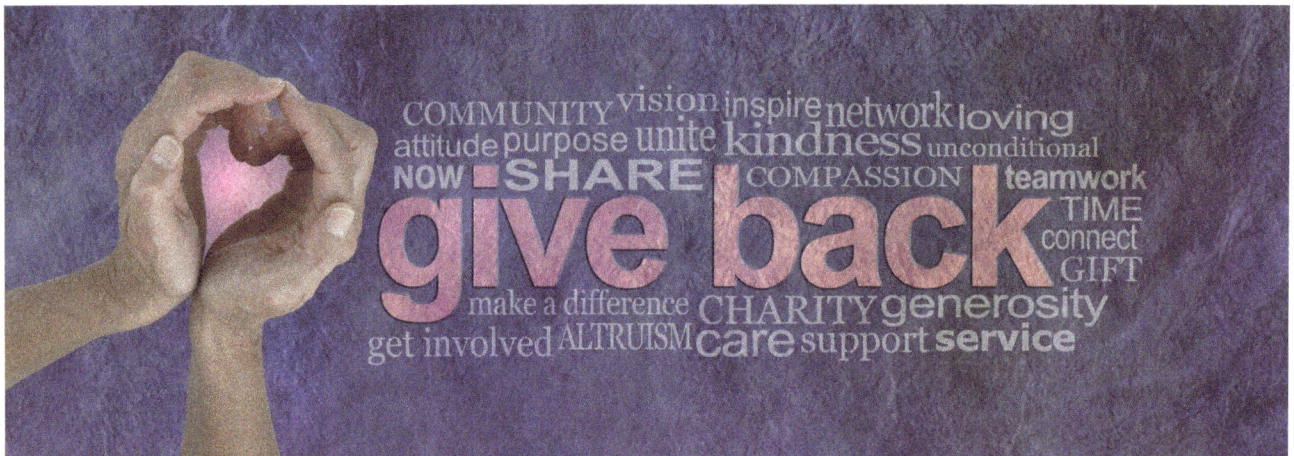

Do you give with strings attached? In other words, do you expect something in return, or do you expect the recipient to "earn" whatever it is you give? Here's why you want to try to change that attitude: whatever judgments you put on your giving are the ones you also put on receiving. Basically, you release yourself from strings and conditions like being worthy or having to repay the gift.

The attitude of an open heart means that you don't just go easy on the other guy, but you also go easier on yourself. We all have strengths, talents, and gifts. It's easier to utilise them when we can accept that we have them. This is easy for some people but quite difficult for others. It isn't false modesty; it's denial. An example most of us are aware of is the extremely good-looking man or woman who says, "I never thought I was handsome/pretty." Don't you wish they could just relax and enjoy such good fortune? The same might be true for you. What are your talents, skills, and positive traits? Claim them, enjoy them and build on them. It will do wonders for your self-esteem and well-being!

Another way to be kind to yourself is to accept and enjoy what someone gives you in the present and remember gifts people have given you in the past. Enjoy the memories and cherish them, free from any negativity. Now, it's true that some gifts you get have strings—that's reality. But recognise that and enjoy the hope that gifts can be given without ulterior motives, and you'll receive those in the future. [96]

In *Recovering From a Broken Heart,* Philip Golabuk explains with great clarity the benefits of keeping an open heart under difficult circumstances:

"When we are unwilling to move in the openness of the heart, we are like a closed hand, which can neither give nor receive. We move through life like a fist—constricted, self-wearying, angry, quick to take offence, ready to lash out. A fist cannot offer support, cannot sustain, cannot feel, cannot express anything but its own hardness. When we accept the present, however, relinquishing criticism and conclusions and simply being with whatever is before us, we find the fist relaxing, the hand opening. Giving and receiving can proceed naturally; we are free to give what is ours to give and receive that which is offered to us as we may wish. At home in both giving and receiving, we no longer need an agenda of winning, taking, outsmarting, of always having to push ourselves toward the next fantasy. All this strategy is replaced by the charm of the moment, which, it might be said, is always giving something and asking us to give something in return. The moment may give the tranquillity of twilight and the soothing music of migrating birds against a slate sky, asking in return that we not let such a moment go unnoticed, unappreciated. It may give us the deep aching that comes when we remember our former partner by a shirt or the way the house smelled when she took fresh cookies from the oven and placed them on a newspaper on the kitchen counter, asking in return that we love this one memory of our partner's sweetness for what it is without having to possess it, that we let our love deepen despite her sadness, perhaps even because of it."

"Missing someone we love has its loveliness, after all. Giving and receiving are part of a life lived from the heart; there is no ownership there, no possessing, no clinging. In this sense, giving and receiving are the natural ebb and flow of letting go and being fully alive. Whether the moment brings happy or sad memories, we can remain wholeheartedly present. We can give and receive without comparing, judging, regretting, without emergency or crisis, without having to do anything at all. We can remain open, even when the mind prompts us to go chasing after the good memories and fills us with anger or remorse over the bad ones. We can let life flow to and from us in the natural dialogue of giving and receiving that contributes greatly to our healing." [97]

## THE SCIENCE BEHIND GIVING

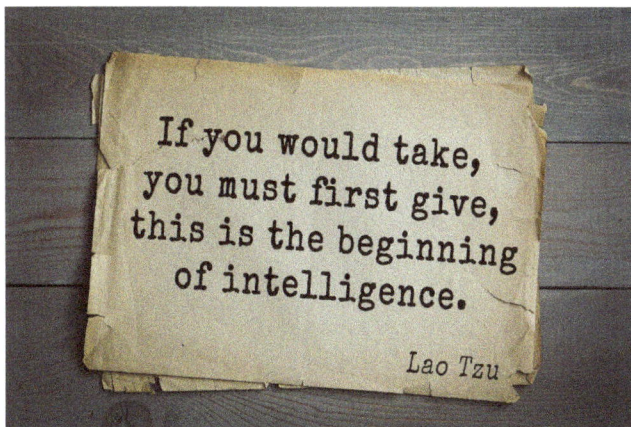

If you would take, you must first give, this is the beginning of intelligence.

Lao Tzu

In *The How of Happiness: A New Approach to Getting the Life You Want,* Sonja Lyubomirsky explains, "I have selected for this book only those activities (from among many) that have been shown to be successful through science, rather than conjecture. What's more, I describe why these strategies work and how precisely they should be implemented to maximise their effectiveness using evidence from the latest research. In every grandmotherly bit of advice lies a kernel of truth. I've chosen the biggest kernels, established what the data show, and sought to determine for whom these truths might work best and how and why. Apply these activities to your own life, and you will harness the promise of the 40 percent solution, for such is the amount of wiggle room you have to remake yourself."[98]

## Acts of Kindness

Lyubomirsky explains, "What scientific research has recently contributed . . . is evidence that practising acts of kindness is not only good for the recipient but also good for the doer. It may be ironic, but being kind and good, even when it's unpleasant or when one expects or receives nothing in return, may also be in the doer's self-interest. This is because being generous and willing to share makes people happy."

Lyubomirsky conducted an experiment in which her students performed five acts of kindness per week over the course of six weeks. The first group performed the acts at any time during the week, while the second group performed all five acts on one day. In this first-ever study of the effects of acts of kindness, the group who spread their acts throughout the week showed no increase in happiness, while the group who performed all the acts in one day reported a great increase. [99]

A second study compared happiness levels of people who performed the same acts of kindness over a ten-week period with those who varied their acts. The group with varied acts of kindness reported an increase in their happiness level, while the group who repeated the same acts reported a dip in their happiness level during the middle of the study with a rise to their original level at the end. Both of these experiments show that variety increases the effect of doing acts of kindness. Performing acts of kindness may result in you "beginning to view yourself as altruistic and compassionate. It can promote a sense of confidence, optimism, and usefulness. It highlights your abilities, resources, and expertise and gives you a feeling of control over your life and increase a sense of meaningfulness and value. It also raised happiness in the second study because the participants recognised definite levels of gratitude in the people they helped.

## Volunteerism

In another study conducted over three years with sixty-seven MS patients and five peer supporters, Lyubomirsky reported that the five peer supporters underwent dramatic changes in their lives as a result of their volunteering. It took the focus off themselves and their problems and caused them to practise more non-judgmental listening and become more open and tolerant of other people as well as giving them a stronger sense of self-esteem and self-acceptance. So, volunteering or community service, while involving a more sustained commitment within an institutional framework, shares many features and benefits with random acts of kindness. [100]

## Gratitude

Dr Lyubomirsky also studied gratitude, or thankfulness, which is the other side of giving/receiving open-heartedness. She defines gratitude not as saying thank you for a gift but "savouring; an antidote to negative emotions, a neutraliser of envy, avarice, hostility, worry, and irritation." She agrees with prominent gratitude researcher and writer, Robert Emma's, that gratitude is "a felt sense of wonder, thankfulness, and appreciation for life."

She set up the studies similarly to the way she had set up the tests for Acts of Kindness and Volunteerism. One group was asked to write five things for which they were grateful one day a week for ten weeks. The control group was asked to think about either five daily hassles or five major events that had occurred during the week. The research found that the participants who expressed gratitude felt more optimistic and more satisfied with their lives than the control group. Even their health was better, with them showing fewer negative symptoms. [101]

Lyubomirsky describes eight benefits of practising gratitude:

1. Gratitude promotes the savouring of positive life experiences. Appreciating your current life keeps you in the present and gives you maximum satisfaction and enjoyment from your existing circumstances.
2. Expressing gratitude increases your self-worth and self-esteem. Many people automatically focus on failures and disappointments. Gratitude refocuses thinking on positive things and can even help unlearn the negative attitude.
3. Gratitude helps people cope with stress and trauma. With regular practise of gratitude, traumatic memories surface less often and are less intense.
4. Grateful people are more likely to help others. They appreciate what they have and become less fixated on acquiring more things.
5. Gratitude can help build social bonds. It can strengthen existing relationships and nurture new ones. It can foster feelings of connectedness.
6. Expressing gratitude can inhibit negative comparisons with others. Being genuinely grateful for what you have means not paying as close attention to what everyone else has.
7. Practising gratitude is incompatible with having negative emotions. It can diminish or even deter negative feelings like anger, bitterness, and greed. It decreases jealousy, fear and defensiveness.
8. Gratitude allows us to enjoy our good experiences for a longer period. We adapt quickly to positive experiences and enjoyment diminishes. Gratitude allows us to savour good experiences, so we enjoy increased well-being for a longer time. [102]

Dr Sonia Lyubomirsky is a pioneer in positive psychology, but she is only one of many researchers. Thousands of studies have been conducted in this field.

A study performed at Harvard in 2009 called "Feeling Good about Giving: The Benefits and Costs of Self-Interested Charitable Behaviour" found that doing good things resulted in benefits for the giver whether the person doing the giving had altruistic intentions or not.

- One study indicated that giving to charity activates the brains regions associated with reward and pleasure. In this study, participants' brains were studied as they discussed giving $100 to charity. They have the choice of giving the entire amount to charity or splitting it between themselves and a charity. Those who decided to give the entire amount activated a part of the brain that responds to a pleasurable experience. Note, this was before they actually donated the money.
- Donating to a not-for-profit charity is actually a double win. You get the good feeling in your brain's pleasure centre, and you also get a deduction when you do your taxes.
- Still another bonus for giving to a charity is that it keeps you involved and informed about what's going on around you. With the availability of the internet, you have easy access to all kinds of information which will help you make an informed decision about the charity you choose. It also will help you become a well-rounded member of your community or society in general, and it may even inspire you to volunteer. [103]

## GIVING TO FAMILY AND FRIENDS

You might think you have nothing to give, but that isn't true, especially when it comes to the people you care about and who care about you. This seemingly smallest thing can have quite an impact. In *The 100 Secrets of Happy People,* Dr David Niven tells us about the power of a smile.

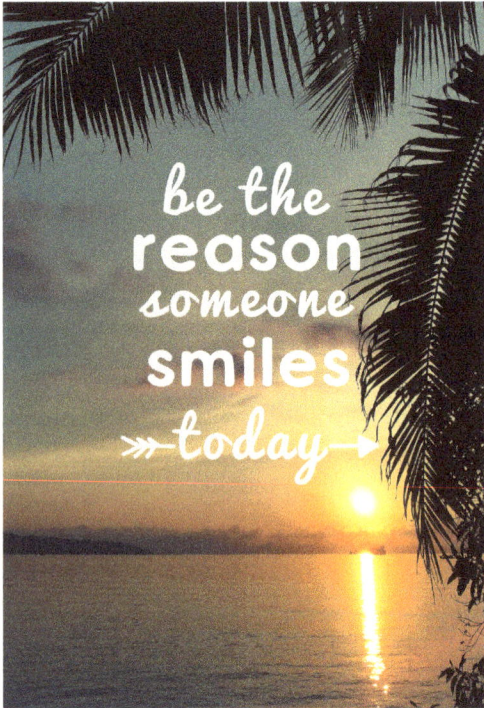

*Smile*

It's been scientifically proven, when you smile, you make other people happy, and that in turn makes you happy. Have you ever tried smiling at a stranger in a meeting or as you walk down the street? Have you noticed how many times they smile back at you? Scientists at the University of California in San Francisco have identified nineteen different kinds of smiles. Each one is capable of communicating a pleasant message that will often be met with a smile in return. In a study of adults of various ages, it was found that subjects mimicked the expressions of those around them—sad faces evoked more sad faces, and smiling faces evoked smiles and happiness.[104]

*Be Agreeable*

Dr David Niven describes an everyday situation any one of us might find ourselves in:

On a Saturday morning, Frank went to play golf with his friend and told his wife, Michelle, that he be back around 2 PM. They played golf, and then he went on to help his friend move some furniture. They took a short lunch break and went back to moving furniture for a while. By the time they were finished, it was 5 PM. Frank had totally forgotten to call Michelle. As he walked through the front door of his house, he was afraid that he might be in trouble, but he apologised and offered to make dinner. Michelle accepted, and they both had a nice evening.

Research shows that having a positive attitude about those around us is among the most important predictors of life satisfaction. Surprisingly, without such attitudes, we are less than half as likely to feel happy.[105]

It's not anyone else's responsibility to keep you happy, just as you can't be responsible for anybody else's happiness. Each person has to do that for themselves, but each one of us is responsible for contributing our share of time and energy to all the relationships that are important to us. It's easy to take people for granted when we're around them a lot of the time, even when we care about them a great deal. One of the most powerful things we can do is listen, really listen, to what the other person is saying and then respond in the most appropriate way. Communication techniques are an asset whether we're talking to a close relative or someone in a social situation, whether it's someone we've known a long time or someone we've just met. Good communication is a highly valuable skill. Here's how to do it.

## GIVING USING THE GIFT OF GOOD COMMUNICATION

Your new mindfulness techniques can play a large part in improving the way you communicate. There are five communication skills (three listening skills and two self-expression skills) in effective communication:

- The Disarming Technique
- Empathy
- Inquiry
- "I feel" statements
- Stroking.

As you read about them, think about how taking a step back, observing the situation, and having some objectivity support these five techniques.

Dr David Burns, a renowned cognitive psychotherapist, describes the five techniques involved in good communication in his classic, *The Feeling Good Handbook*. He says that "More than anything else, people want to be cared about and appreciated. What we fear the most is being rejected or put down or judged. Therefore, I always try to express positive regard for the other person, even in the heat of battle. I try to let them know that I respect them and that they're important to me. This can alleviate unspoken fears that someone is going to get rejected. Burns incorporates this approach into the five techniques.

## 1. The Disarming Technique

This technique is difficult but powerful, especially if it's a situation where you feel you are being criticised or attacked. It consists of trying to find a grain of truth in what the other person is saying even when you think what they are saying is completely wrong, unreasonable, irrational, or unfair. You need to resist the urge to argue or defend yourself so that in the end, you can both feel like winners.

Here's an example: supposing your spouse says to you, "You're always late, and I'm sick of waiting for you." What could you say to disarm her? You could say something like, "It's true. I am late, and you have the right to be angry." Do you see how this works to disarm her? When you admit that you're late, your spouse feels listened to and respected. On the other hand, if you get defensive and start making excuses, your spouse might become even more irate.

You need to be genuine when you're using this technique, or it won't work. But you should usually be able to find something valid to agree about. When that happens, the other person will be more inclined to listen to you. You are often likely to be able to win them over to your point of view because you understand where they're coming from. You're no longer on opposite sides, each defending your own point of view; instead, you're building a relationship. Once they see you respect them, they will soften and acknowledge your feelings and ideas.

## 2. Empathy

Empathy means that you try to put yourself in the other person's shoes and understand what he/she is thinking. Repeat what the other person is saying, so they know you understand, but don't say it sarcastically or defensively. Try to be genuinely curious. Then acknowledge the feelings they might have and ask a question to see if you are reading his/her emotions correctly. Notice their body language—are they tense or hurt or angry? Accept the other person's feelings without being hostile or critical or defensive. This shows that you are open to hearing what they have to say.

## 3. Inquiry

Inquiry means the use of gentle, probing questions to learn more about what the other person is thinking and feeling. Most people have trouble expressing angry feelings. The inquiry technique helps to get the other person's feelings out in the open, so you know how things stand. This is good because often when people deny their feelings, they act them out instead of expressing them, and this can be destructive for both parties. An effective way to avoid this is to ask the other person to tell you more about his negative feelings. Then ask directly what you did or said to cause the hurt feelings. When they tell you, don't get defensive. Find some truth in what they have to say. Be respectful, not challenging or sarcastic. Don't be afraid of the other person expressing anger. If handled right, you can diffuse the anger which might have built if it remained unexpressed.

## 4. "I feel" Statements.

An "I feel" statement is a technique you used to express yourself. This diffuses a situation because instead of accusing the other person with statements like, "You're wrong" or "You don't know what you're talking about," you're saying what you feel. This is a simple but powerful technique. Since you're not being critical or judgmental about what the other person is saying, you are free to express what you are feeling, whether your feelings are negative or positive.

## 5. Stroking

Many people are quite afraid of expressing anger because they believe that if they do, the other person won't care for them anymore. People are immensely afraid of being put down, rejected, or judged. Stroking lets the other person know that even though you disagree about an issue, you still have high regard for her. Let her know that even though you disagree with her in this instance about something she's thinking or feeling, you still like and respect her and your goal is to work out the issue. Don't ever make it a personal attack. Stick with the issue that's being discussed. That's the only way to make headway.

Can you see how mindfulness and communication techniques go hand-in-hand? Mindfulness gives you the breathing space to be objective, and communication techniques give you the skills to build successful relationships of all kinds.[106]

## VOLUNTEERING

Volunteering England, part of the National Council for Voluntary Organisations (NCVO), reports that more than 20 million people across the UK donate more than 100 million hours to their community. This amounts to an estimated economic value of more than L40 billion.

Volunteering England commissioned the University of Wales to do a study on the effects of volunteering on volunteers. The results showed that the volunteers often benefited as much as the people they were helping. The research showed benefits that included.

- Longer life expectancy compared to non-volunteers
- Greater ability for volunteers to come to terms with their own illnesses and better performance in their own daily lives

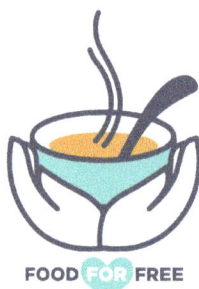

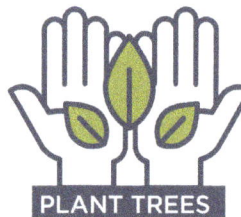

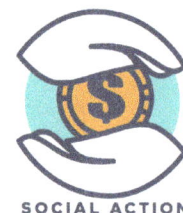

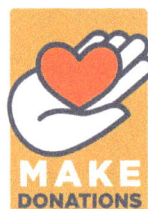

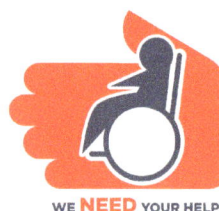

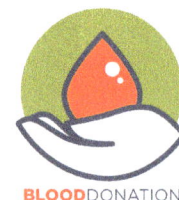

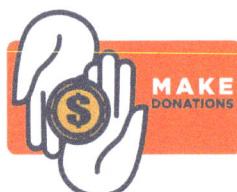

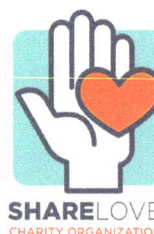

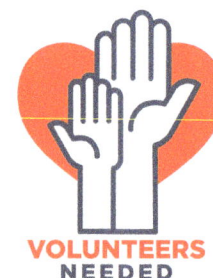

- Better behaviour in their own lives. For instance, volunteers who worked in non-smoking wards often gave up smoking; college students who volunteered often drank less than non-volunteering college students
- Improved family relationships for older volunteers because volunteering gave them a sense of being more independent and less reliant on their family
- Volunteers felt better integrated into society because of meeting people through volunteering
- Better self-esteem and a greater sense of purpose through the work they did as volunteers
- A better outlook on their own health than non-volunteers.

Surprisingly perhaps, the research revealed benefits for the patients the volunteers worked with. These benefits included

- Increased self-esteem and confidence: volunteers can act as mediators, improving the relationship between the hospital staff and patient, thus improving everyone's attitude
- Better social interaction, integration and support: patients saw volunteers as peers and were more inclined to converse with them
- Reduced burden on carers: support from volunteers assisted carers and allowed them to perform their caring duties more effectively
- Decreased anxiety: patients who were about to go through a procedure were less anxious when they could talk to a volunteer who had had the same procedure.
- Longer survival time for hospice patients: surprising but true, hospice patients who had visits from volunteers lived quite a bit longer than those who didn't
- An increase in breastfeeding and childhood immunisation: volunteers provided help to young or disadvantaged mothers by educating them about breastfeeding and vaccinations as well as influencing how often children were taken for their standard checkups
- Improved clinic attendance and taking of their medications: having a volunteer who can act as a mediator during clinic appointments can improve the chances of a patient correctly following up with medication and appointments. [107]

Everything considered, volunteering is a win-win for volunteers and patients alike.

## How To Volunteer

So, does volunteering sound like something that you would be interested in? If so, the first thing you need to do is decide what kind of volunteering would be good for you. Think about the type of organisation you might like, the activities you'd like to get involved in, and how much time you might have to spend. There are all kinds of volunteering positions, and you can spend as little as a lunch hour or a lot more time if you choose.

Sometimes volunteer work is supported by employers. Some employers set up different types of volunteering programs, while other employers offer time off for employees to do their own projects. Check with your employer. If he doesn't have one already, you might suggest one or even help to set one up.

You might have a personal interest in the issue you'd like to volunteer for. You might have a health problem yourself or a family member or friend with a problem that inspires you to volunteer your time to work or to fundraise.

A good way to find out about volunteering opportunities in your area is to contact your local NHS organisation. You could search your local NHS website for more information about places to volunteer, or you could go to your local library. Your librarian would be able to help you.

An innovative way to participate in volunteering is to use a time bank. This allows you to offer your skills in return for credit, which you can then use to buy someone else's services. For instance, you could tutor someone for three hours and receive three hours of language lessons in return. Visit the Time Banking UK website (www.timebanking.org) to learn more.

You might be interested in contacting the following national organisations for details on volunteering:

### CSV (Community Service Volunteers)

CSV was founded to encourage young people aged 16 to 35 to volunteer. Possible opportunities include work on environmental projects, helping children to read and supporting people who are unwell and unable to carry out day-to-day tasks. You could also get involved with health-focused projects, open to people of all ages on a part-time or full-time basis. Visit the www.csv.org.uk to find something that suits you.

### Do-it

Do-it is the only national database of volunteering opportunities in the UK. The www.do-it.org.uk allows you to search volunteering opportunities by area of interest and postcode.

### Volunteering England

Volunteering England is an independent agency with links to national charities, voluntary agencies, arts organisations, local community projects and NHS trusts. On the website, www.volunteeringengland.org you can locate centres that provide information on volunteering opportunities in your area and that can also help match you to vacancies.[108]

## GIVE BACK TO YOUR COMMUNITY

Here are some ideas for specific ways you could choose to volunteer:

### Make New Friends At The Shelter

Animal shelters are almost always looking for extra help and volunteers. While there might be some unglamorous tasks on occasion, you'll also get to spend some quality time with really loving, adorable animals.

### Organise A Clothing Sale

If you enjoy fashion, consider organising a clothing sale. Ask people in your community to donate new or gently used clothing and accessories, and re-label them for reasonable resale prices. Donate all the proceeds from the sale to a local charity—like a soup kitchen or animal shelter—then donate any of the remaining un-purchased clothes to a local shelter.

### Go Green At The Community Garden

Love gardening? Consider taking up a plot at the community garden or volunteering to help maintain the unclaimed or common areas. No community garden in your town? What a great project for you and your neighbours to start!

### Get Your Arts and Crafts On A Local Theatre

If you like theatre, you may be able to find volunteer work you'll enjoy at a community theatre or school. Tell them your speciality and ask if they have any sets that need painting, costumes that need sewing or props that need building.

### Share Your Skills

There are lots of places looking for volunteers to help with activities for kids—schools, after-school care programs, day care centres, camps, church groups, the YMCA, mentorship programs and more. Even if you don't think you're particularly talented, you may be able to help children learn to paint a picture, ride a bike, make a free throw, fold origami, jump rope, grow a plant, braid hair and more. It just takes a phone call and a little patience.

### Double Your Dessert

Next time you're baking for a family or work event, consider doubling your batch and bringing the extras to a local police station, veteran club, senior home or soup kitchen There are plenty of places that will appreciate your skills!

### Share Your Smarts

We've all got something we're good at, and if you're lucky enough to be good at long division or skilled in Spanish conjugations, consider sharing your smarts with local students. Many schools and after-school programs would be happy to take on a volunteer to help students improve.

### Visit Local Seniors

Senior Centres will almost always take volunteers, and sometimes you don't have to do anything other than say hello and listen to some pretty cool stories. But you can also read, play cards, dance, run an art class, give residents manicures—whatever!

### Boost Careers As A Resume Editor

Got a way with words or a sharp eye for detail? Consider helping your fellow residents with their careers by volunteering as a resume editor. See if local high schools, transitional houses, shelters or veteran assistance programs might be interested in having you come in and offer a workshop. You might even be able to get a local business to donate resume paper. [109]

Important note: Are you one of those people who loves to give but is not comfortable when it comes to receiving anything, even something small like a compliment? Lots of people feel that way. But the truth is that that attitude denies other people the joy of giving to you, and other people like giving, too! If you take a mindful minute to consider that receiving will give both you and the giver joy, you'll be comfortable with it.

# PUTTING IDEAS INTO PRACTISE

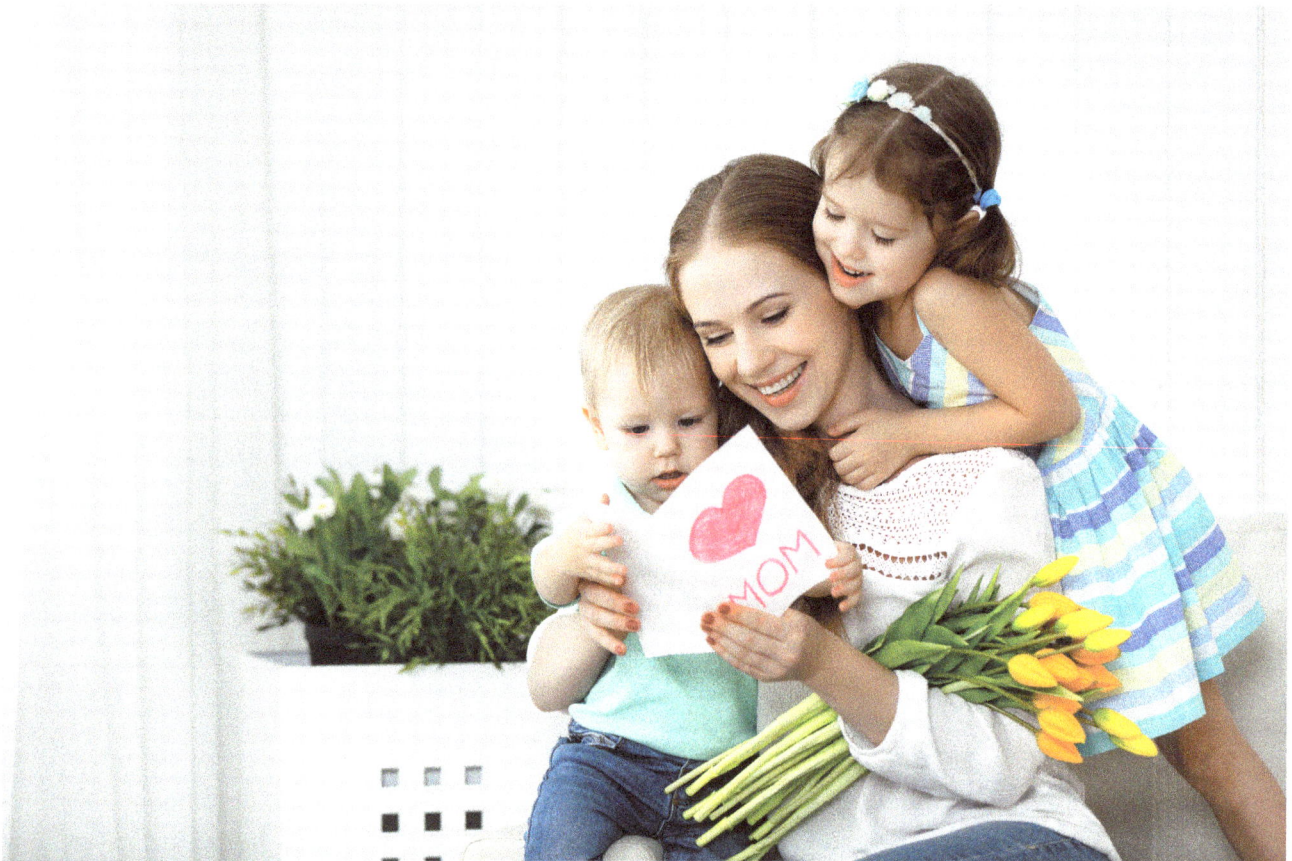

Do these exercises this week or in the near future:

1. Leave a gift or an amount that you can afford, but that is still meaningful to you (£1, £10, £100—whatever amount is significant to you) in a nursing home or a place where people can really do with some cheering up. Leave it anonymously. The point is to try to reserve judgment about who picks it up. This is an exercise about you practising letting go of the strings when you give. Also, watch how the people receive it. Look at their faces. Are they surprised and happy?

2. Make double portions of a casserole or another comfort food and bring it to a new neighbour, an elderly neighbour, or one with health problems. We all have comfort foods to choose from, right? It could be cake, rice pudding and sweet potatoes, and so on. (Make it something you can cook well, of course!) Get to know a little about the person when you bring over the food. Many times, these days, we don't know even our closest neighbours. Maybe it will be the start of a friendship.

3. Appreciate a spouse or other family member and express it. Familiarity can lead to taking each other for granted. Even the most stoic among us, people who don't seem to need anything, really appreciate some recognition and a compliment from time to time. It's easy to get irritated by the other person's faults—but make it a point to remember their good qualities like their patience or the way they support you. Appreciating the other person isn't only good for him. It gives you joy as well.

4. Give a motivational book or a CD to a friend who seems to be a little down or who has experienced a setback. Talk to the person about what's wrong. If he/she might benefit from some professional counselling, suggest it. Is there a group they might join that they could benefit from? Let them know.

Go for a walk with together or suggest an outing for the two of you. It might matter more than you know.

5. Write a thank-you note or a sincere email to someone you value who has helped you in the past. Let them know that you remember and appreciate them. Include an inspirational quote or a funny cartoon to brighten their day.

Here's what the folks at the Five Ways to Wellness app are doing:

## EXAMPLES OF HOW TO GIVE

"I was outside when I noticed my neighbour looking like she was struggling with carrying packages. I offered to take them into her back garden for her, and she agreed, she was ever so grateful and invited me in for coffee. We got chatting, and she told me how she was a painter and showed me some of the pictures she had painted. I was very impressed with one, and she sold it to me half price! Now my neighbour and I are good friends."

*"We make a living by what we get. We make a life by what we give."*
—Winston Churchill

# THE CRITICAL HALF WAY TO WELL-BEING

*"The key difference between "5 and 1/2 ways to well-being" and "5 ways to well-being" is the difference between success and failure because taking massive action leads to consistent results for lifelong vitality, health and happiness"*
—Ruben Seetharamdoo

Critical? Yes, this chapter is critical because even when you know what to change and how to change it, it won't do you much good without being able to sustain your motivation to do so. Have you ever made a New Year's resolution or know someone who has? Then you know that there comes a point where you're ready to quit—and probably do. The dynamics in New Year's resolutions are the same ones that could sabotage your journey to well-being, so let's take a good look at what goes on with New Year's resolutions.

## WHY DO RESOLUTIONS FAIL?

The top 10 New Year's resolutions recently were:

1.  Lose weight
2.  Get organised
3.  Spend less, save more
4.  Enjoy life to the fullest
5.  Stay fit and healthy
6.  Learn something exciting
7.  Quit smoking
8.  Help others in their dreams
9.  Fall in love
10. Spend more time with family.

This list might include some of the things you have in mind to increase your well-being, right? Then you might be interested in the percentage of people who actually achieve their resolution – it's 8%! Little by little, people fall by the wayside. Here's the length of time they were able to keep their resolutions:

| | |
|---|---|
| Resolution maintained through the first week | 75% |
| Resolution kept for two weeks | 71% |
| Resolutions kept past one month | 64% |
| Resolutions kept past six months | 46% |
| Resolutions successful at the two-year point | 8%[110] |

The reasons people gave for not keeping their resolutions is especially interesting to us in our quest for increased well-being. Here's the list:

*   Feeling a lack of personal control
*   Excessive stress
*   Social pressure
*   Interpersonal conflict.[111]

Do you recognise the emotional component in each one of these reasons for not succeeding at keeping New Year's resolutions? The study noted that self-blame and criticism were especially strong in people who were unable to keep their resolutions. So what does that tell us about why we quit before we fulfil our dreams and goals? Simply put, we get frustrated. In one way or another, our negative emotions get the best of us. This is especially sad since, as we've learned in previous chapters, our

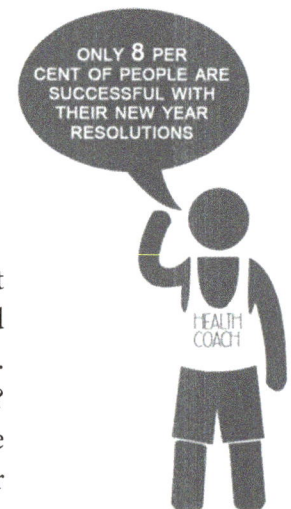

ONLY **8** PER CENT OF PEOPLE ARE SUCCESSFUL WITH THEIR NEW YEAR RESOLUTIONS

HEALTH COACH

emotions are more often than not based on irrational thinking—regrets and anger about the past and worry about the future—that overwhelms us.

It doesn't have to be that way.

We have the knowledge, the skills, the understanding, the science, and even a blueprint to successfully pursue happiness as we've never been able to before. And you can see from reading the previous chapters that it isn't that hard. The key is simple awareness and willingness to move toward a more mindful attitude about how we live our everyday lives.

The rest of this chapter will give you a blueprint for handling negative emotions that frustrate us and kill our motivation and some techniques for dealing with common problems that arise on the road to increased well-being.

## BLUEPRINT FOR WELL-BEING

Remember the old joke, "Why are you beating your head against the wall?" Answer: "Because it feels so good when I stop." Well, in David Burns' book, *The Feeling Good Handbook,* he tells us in easy-to-understand language how to improve our mental health. Now, if you have a severe mental health issue, you should always seek professional help. But when it comes to everyday mental well-being, Burns' book is a gold mine. In it, he gives us a succinct blueprint that he calls "The Four Steps to Happiness." It consists of four simple steps:

1.  Identify the problem
2.  Notice your negative feelings
3.  Use Burns' triple column technique
4.  Acknowledge the outcome.

Here's his explanation of the technique:

STEP ONE — Identify the upsetting situation. Describe the event or problem that's upsetting you. Who (or what) are you feeling unhappy about?

STEP TWO — Record your negative feelings. How do you feel about the upsetting situation? Use words like sad, angry, anxious, guilty, frustrated, hopeless. Rate each negative feeling on a scale from 1 (for the least) to 100 (for the most).

STEP THREE — use the triple column technique. Tune in to the negative thoughts that are associated with these feelings. What are you saying to yourself about the problem? Record these thoughts in the Automatic Thoughts column and record how much you believe each one between 0 (not at all) and 100 (completely). After you identify the distortions in these thoughts, substitute rational responses in the right-hand column and record how much you believe each one between 0 (not at all) and 100 (completely). Make sure that your rational responses are convincing, valid statements that invalidate your Automatic Thoughts.

STEP FOUR — Indicate how much you now believe each Automatic Thought between 0 and 100. Once your belief in these thoughts is greatly reduced, indicate how much better you feel. [112]

You could dedicate a portion of your journal or open a new file on your computer and call it The Daily Mood Log (as Burns does). Then, you would write down Step One and describe the upsetting event. Then, write down Step Two and record your negative feelings along with you rating for them. (Use the words Burns suggests or other words that come to mind.) Next, make three columns: Automatic Thoughts, Distortions, and Rational Responses. Write down the thoughts and rate them, identify the distortions, write down more rational thoughts and rate them.

Do you see how the system can be effective? Once you begin to use this consistently in response to your thoughts, you might not need to write them down. In fact, using this system could very well become a new habit for you.

Remember the various types of thinking errors we discussed in the previous chapter ("Types of Thinking Errors and Examples by Dr Gary Emery)? You could use those to help you identify your distortions in thinking.

## COGNITIVE DISTORTIONS CHECKLIST

In addition, Dr Burns created a checklist similar to Emery's but different in some important ways. It's brief but quite valuable for helping to define thinking errors. Here it is:

### Checklist Of Cognitive Distortions

1.  All or nothing thinking: You look at things in absolute, black and white categories.
2.  Overgeneralisation: You view a negative event as a never-ending pattern of defeat.
3.  Mental filter: You dwell on the negatives and ignore the positives.
4.  Discounting the positives: You insist that your accomplishments or positive qualities "don't count."
5.  Jumping to conclusions: (A) Mind reading: you assume that people are reacting negatively to you when there's no definite evidence for this; (B) Fortune-telling: you arbitrarily predict that things will turn out badly.
6.  Magnification or minimisation: You blow things way up out of a portion, or you shrink their importance inappropriately.
7.  Emotional reasoning: You reason from how you feel: "I feel like an idiot, so I really must be one." Or "I don't feel like doing this, so I'll put it off."
8.  "Should statements": You criticise yourself or other people with "shoulds" or "shouldn'ts" "musts," "oughts," and "have tos" are similar offenders.
9.  Labelling: You identify with your shortcomings. Instead of saying," I made a mistake," you tell yourself," I'm a jerk," or" a fool," or" a loser."
10. Personalisation and blame: You blame yourself for something you weren't entirely responsible for, or you blame other people and overlooked ways that your own attitudes and behaviour might contribute to a problem.[113]

### Straight Thinking

Now for some solutions! Dr Burns puts it this way, "When you feel bad, you are thinking about things in a negative way." I don't think you can put it more clearly or more simply than that. And the solution lies in the statement of the problem. If our negative thinking is making us feel bad, then switching that negative thinking to positive thinking will make us feel good. Burns gives us some simple, effective techniques for, as he calls it, "untwisting our thinking."

- Identify the Distortion. Write down your negative thoughts so you can see which of the ten cognitive distortions you're involved in. This will make it easier to think about the problem in a more positive and realistic way.

- Examine the Evidence. Instead of assuming that your negative thought is true, examine the actual evidence for it. For example, if you feel that you never do anything right, you could list several things you have done successfully.
- The Double Standard Method. Instead of putting yourself down in a harsh, condemning way, talk to yourself in the same compassionate way you would talk to a friend with a similar problem.
- The Experimental Technique. Do an experiment to test the validity of your negative thought. For example, if, during an episode of panic, you become terrified that you're about to die the architect, you could jog or run up and down several flights of stairs. This will prove that your heart is healthy and strong.
- Thinking in Shades of Grey. With this is a draft, the effects can be illuminating. Instead of thinking about your problems in all or nothing extremes, evaluate, things on a range from 0 to 100. When things don't work out as well as you hoped, think about the experience as a partial success rather than a complete failure. See what you can learn from the situation.
- The Survey Method. Ask people questions to find out if your thoughts and attitudes a realistic. For example, if you believe that public speaking anxiety is abnormal and shameful, ask several friends if they ever felt nervous before they gave a talk.
- Define Terms. When you label yourself "inferior" or "a fool" or "loser," ask, "what is the definition of 'a fool'?" You will feel better when you see that there is no such thing as a "fool" or "loser."
- The Semantic Method. Simply substitute language that is less colourful and emotionally loaded. This method is helpful for "should statements." Instead of telling yourself. "I shouldn't have made that mistake," you can say, "it would be better if I hadn't made that mistake."
- Re-attribution. Instead of automatically assuming that you are "bad" and blaming yourself entirely for a problem, think about the many factors that may have contributed to it. Focus on solving the problem. Instead of using all your energy blaming yourself and feeling guilty.
- Cost-Benefit Analysis. List the advantages and disadvantages of a feeling (like getting angry when your plane is late) a negative thought (like, "No matter how hard I try, I always screw up"), or a behaviour pattern (like overeating and lying around in bed when you're depressed). You can also use the Cost-Benefit Analysis to modify self-defeating beliefs such as, "I must always try to be perfect." [114]

Can you see the great power you have when you take one mindful minute to objectively look at what you're thinking and reframe it from negative to positive? It's the most powerful thing in the world; you know how to do it, and I hope you take advantage of it because it works.

### Some Good Tips For Staying On Course

Skillful mindfulness plus knowledge about handling specific troublesome thoughts and emotions will prepare you for those thoughts and emotions when they come up. You will begin to experience the satisfaction of feeling in charge of your life. As you get more done, you will have order where you used to have chaos. You will know what you want, and you will want to move ahead to get it. Once you begin to complete your dreams and goals one at a time, you will have renewed confidence in your ability to succeed.

But even when you have the best of intentions, you might encounter some of these common stumbling blocks:

### Unstable Mindset

Question: What's the best mindset to ensure that I will keep moving toward my goals?

The participants in the New Year's resolutions study expressed lack of personal control, excessive stress, social pressure, and interpersonal conflict as reasons for giving up on their resolutions. We can learn a few things from them.

First, they probably didn't know about or didn't practise mindfulness. If they did, they would have understood that these problems might come up even before they made their resolutions or would have known how to handle the problems when they came up.

Second, they were not 100% committed to the resolutions they made. That's fine, but in reality, if we want to increase some aspect of our well-being, we need to commit to it in the face of obstacles including social pressure from others. Practising mindfulness means that we are responsible for everything that is going on in our lives. A better way to handle "social pressure" and "interpersonal conflict" is to use the communication skills we learned in a previous chapter so that others in our lives understand our goals and their importance to us.

Third, the goal of increasing well-being is to get better—not to quit because we haven't reached perfection due to "lack of personal control." The key is to be flexible and adjust to circumstances, but not to give up entirely. The questions to ask are, "Am I improving?" and "Is there a way to adjust my circumstances so that I can achieve my goal?" Once again, stepping back, taking a breath, and assessing the situation objectively works wonders.

## Fuzzy Goals

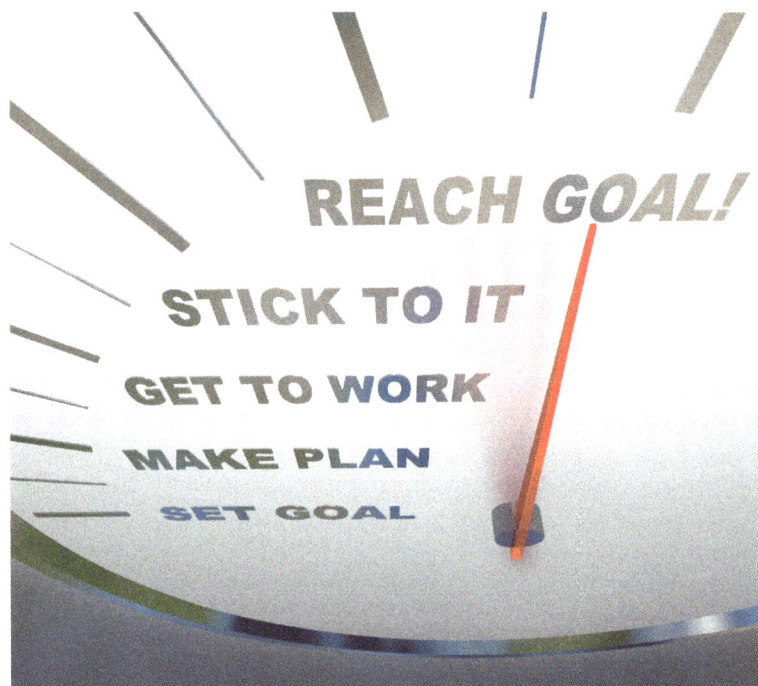

Question: How do I create clear, realistic, achievable goals?

I have a feeling that the failure rate of people who make New Year's resolutions is so high because they're operating from "shoulds" instead of "musts." In other words, they think they should lose weight or they should get organised, and they're probably right, but they don't really want to. They're operating out of two opposing desires, so it makes perfect sense that they would sabotage themselves. It isn't a conscious thing, but it's real and probably inevitable. It's no wonder that the two top reasons for quitting New Year's resolutions lack the personal control and excessive stress. An internal battle of wills is quite stressful. The solution? A few mindful minutes when you ask yourself, "What is it that I really want?" Based on your answer, you may decide to drop the project you're working on, but the good news is that your stress will be gone, and you'll be able to move onto another project you genuinely want to tackle.

Once we decided on the goals we really want to achieve, a few more obstacles might arise. A common one is a frustration at not seeing progress as quickly as we expected to. This is a critical juncture because it's the point where a lot of people quit. They feel they made a mistake and the goal is unreachable. They begin to feel that it's all too hard and they're not competent enough to do it.

This is once again the time for a few mindful minutes. It's time to take a look, not at the goal, but at the way you're going about achieving it. There's no point in continuing to take actions that are not giving you the results you want. This is the time to tweak your plan, change your actions, and assess the new results. You may have to repeat this process several times along the way until you successfully reach your goal.

## Wavering Motivation

Question: How can I keep my motivation strong in the face of obstacles?

Motivation is an area where mindfulness can really shine. So many obstacles can get in the way of us consistently pursuing increased well-being. And it only takes a temporary lack of motivation for us to give up on the whole thing. That's a shame because if we only take a minute to think about it, we have so many ways to get our enthusiasm back.

First, you need to be sure that your priorities haven't changed. Whatever your original goal was, is it still important to you? For instance, do you still want a boyfriend, or is it time to move on? Is getting healthy still worth the effort? It's a lot of work—do you even still want a college degree? If your honest answer to those things is no, the only thing you might succeed in doing is making yourself miserable. It's a good idea to reassess your goals every six months or so at least.

If the answer is yes and you're still interested in achieving those goals, the next question is, "Am I fulfilling my goals or someone else's?" We grow up trying to please our parents; we want to make them happy. Often, we assume that the goals they have for us are best for us. But if they're not the goals we truly want for ourselves, we won't be happy. It's a sad thing that many people spend their entire lives achieving other people's goals. If there's ever a time to practise mindfulness, it's when you are looking at your goals to be sure that they are authentically yours.

Now that you've established that your goals haven't changed and they are your authentic goals, let's take a look at what motivates you as a person. Are you more motivated by moving toward pleasure or avoiding pain? Knowing the answer to that question can increase your motivation. So, which means more you? The fear of missing a deadline or the pleasure of taking two days off after you've made your deadline? One way you can find out is to take a sheet of paper and write down all the benefits of taking action versus all the negative outcomes of not taking action. One side will probably jump out at you. Whichever one does, keep that front and centre in your mind as your motivation.

Next, let's whip your self-talk into shape. If your motivation is flagging, you must be making negative statements in your mind about what you're doing. The key here is to recognise those statements and to talk back to them. Many times, we are so used to our own negative statements that we don't even hear them. That's when they can run riot. They could be saying things to you like, "This is never going to work. I'm missing out on so many good times, and I'll still never save enough for a car" or "I'll never be thin. I've missed a lot of good meals for nothing." And on and on. This is when you step in and talk back to that voice. For instance, "It's only been a month, and I have already saved an extra £60 for the car. In another six months I'll have a down payment" or "Five pounds is a good start. I'm going to stick with it." Whatever it is, give yourself credit for your hard work to this point and realise that if you persist with it, you will meet your goal. If it helps you, you could write down all your negative thoughts on one side in your journal and all your positive answers to those thoughts on the other side.

Another tactic to improve motivation is to take a break. If you've been working at your goal consistently for a period of time, no matter how much you want it, it might be getting a little tedious and boring. Take a day off. A change of pace can be very effective. For instance, if you've been sticking to a strict diet for a month, a cheat day when you eat anything that you want could get you back to your diet the next day with enthusiasm. The same thing goes for going to the gym. You do need to know yourself, however. It could get you off your diet or out of the gym permanently, and we don't want that.

Still another effective tactic to increase your motivation is to procrastinate deliberately. It's a variation on the last tactic. It gives you a change of pace while you're building up the enthusiasm to get back to your main task. This can work quite effectively. I know a writer who loves to write but has trouble doing it on a consistent schedule. Her solution is to clean her house for a certain period of time and then get down to writing. She hasn't wasted her time because she has a clean house, and the cleaning helped her get into the mood to write. It's sort of a win-win for her.

Other people find it quite effective to schedule a task for a specific amount of time and to work on it during that time only. That way, they are free to do whatever they want with the rest of their time without feeling guilty that they're procrastinating.

When it comes to a lack of motivation, practising mindfulness gives you great flexibility because you've become skilled at looking at a problem from many different angles. If one solution doesn't work for you, you'll think of another one.

## FEAR OF FAILURE

Question: How can I combat a feeling that I'm going to fail at achieving my goals?

The first thing to remember is that we all sometimes fail at some things. Remember Edison and the light bulb. When asked how he felt about failing 10,000 times, he said,

"I'm 10,000 times closer to inventing the light bulb." That's a perfect example of a good attitude about failure for two reasons: Edison doesn't let the failures define him as a person; in other words, a failure in his business does not mean he's a failure. Second, he sees each failure as a learning experience that brings him closer to ultimate success.

So, the question to ask yourself is, "Why am I feeling so afraid?" People who are afraid of failure often base their self-esteem on their accomplishments. They fear that failure in anything could mean the loss of love and respect from others as well as the loss of their own self-esteem. Because they place so much importance on succeeding, they can't risk doing anything at all.

They magnify a failure into a catastrophe, representing not just failure of one thing, but everything in their lives. By practising mindful thinking, we can see that failure in one thing is not failure in everything. For instance, if I set a goal to lose five pounds in two weeks and I only lose 3 pounds, I didn't reach my goal, but I'm three pounds closer to my ultimate weight loss goal. And it's only one aspect of my life. I'm on the right track, and I'll lose the other two pounds and more in time. When looked at that way, which is the correct way to look at it, it's not really a failure at all.

If you find yourself afraid to take action because you might fail, ask yourself if you're placing too much importance on that one task. If so, adjust your attitude about the consequences and take action.

Remember too that you're trying to increase your well-being which means you happiness. If an obstacle to that shows up in the form of perfectionism, that's a good thing because you are forced to realise that perfectionism is a weakness you need to work on. Many of us were raised with the belief that we should always try to do things perfectly and be "the best." Of course, that's an impossible demand to live up to. We can't change what we can't see. But now that we see we have a perfectionistic attitude, we can begin to lighten up on ourselves.

High standards are fine, but not when they paralyse you. There's a difference between perfectionism and healthy pursuit of our best self. Healthy personal growth is joyful, and you're enthusiastic about pursuing it. When you make progress, you have a sense of accomplishment even if you haven't reached your initial target. Your self-esteem is not at risk, and you're not afraid to fail because it's an opportunity for growth. You realise that if other people think less of you because of this "failure," they are the ones perceiving the situation incorrectly.[115]

## FEAR OF SUCCESS

Question: Something is holding me back, but I don't know what it is. What is a fear of success, anyway?

Now, that is a VERY interesting question and one you need to answer because anything you do to increase your well-being is moving toward success. So, the answer is that it's not success per se that we fear—it is change. Change is anything we do that we're not accustomed to doing. If I want to increase my well-being by 10%, just as an example, I will have to change what I do by 10%. Change is scary for human beings even when the change will mean improvement. It just is.

Okay then, the next question you might ask is, "If change is so scary, why would I want to do it?" Another good question, and one with a fascinating answer. Do you know when human beings are happiest? It's not when they are doing the things that they are very familiar with. And it's not when they are doing things that are completely unfamiliar to them. It's the sweet spot right in the middle. It's when they're familiar with most of the task or the situation (whatever it is) and are being challenged just a bit to learn something new. Really. Numerous studies have shown this. And that's why we're both afraid of change and desire it at the same time. And that's why we're afraid of success.

That sets up a bit of a conundrum, doesn't it? You bet. Luckily, though, we have some tools to deal with it. Once again, Dr David Burns gets credit. First, he explains the difference between very successful people and others, and it really comes down to successful people having a more realistic attitude about what it takes to succeed.

Successful people understand that motivation doesn't come first—productive action does. You have to prime the pump by getting started whether you feel like it or not. Once you have begun to succeed at something, it will usually encourage you to do even more. A second very important difference between successful people and others is that they assume that life will be frustrating and that there will be failures and obstacles on the road to success. Since they assume this, it doesn't throw them for a loop when the obstacles arrive. They simply persist, with more determination and commitment. [116]

Many people assume that successful people have qualities that make success easy for them. It isn't true. They're simply working from a different model than other people. So, it isn't due to a character defect or anything like that when we don't achieve things easily. Yet, it's this incorrect belief that often causes people to quit.

Burns created a model named "prescription for procrastinators," which he claims has caused many people to become more productive and successful. It consists of five steps that will help you to achieve your goals:

## PRESCRIPTION FOR PROCRASTINATORS

1. Cost-Benefit Analysis: ask yourself why you're procrastinating (putting off whatever it is that you should do). List the advantages and disadvantages of getting started today. Once you analyse all the advantages and disadvantages, you will decide the project isn't worth doing after all, or you will go on to the next step.

2.  Make a Plan: if you have decided that the advantages outweigh the disadvantages, write down a specific time when you will start the project. Then list any problems or obstacles that might get in the way of you beginning the project. Finally, write down the solutions to those problems next to the problems.

3.  Make the Job Easy — Make your goals achievable and realistic. Break down your task step-by-step, so that's clearly doable. Don't schedule more than you can do realistically in any time period. It's a good idea to break things down into 15-minute periods of work since you can stick with even an unpleasant task for a short period of time.

4.  Think Positively: At this point, take a good look at your thoughts. Are they negative? Write them down. It helps you to face them and, in all likelihood, see that they are unrealistic. Talk back to the negative thoughts with some positive self-talk. Write down your positive thoughts across from the negative thoughts.

5.  Give yourself credit for the things you've accomplished instead of berating yourself because you haven't done enough. [117]

With mindfulness, the knowledge that we all fear change and this five-step plan, you should be on your way to resolving your fear of success.

Finally, we all have a day once in a while when we just don't want to make an effort. Sounds human to me. It shouldn't be work. It should be something you enjoy. So, don't be afraid to take a day off. Your journey to well-being is long term. You'll enjoy it more when you get back to it.

## PUTTING IDEAS INTO PRACTISE

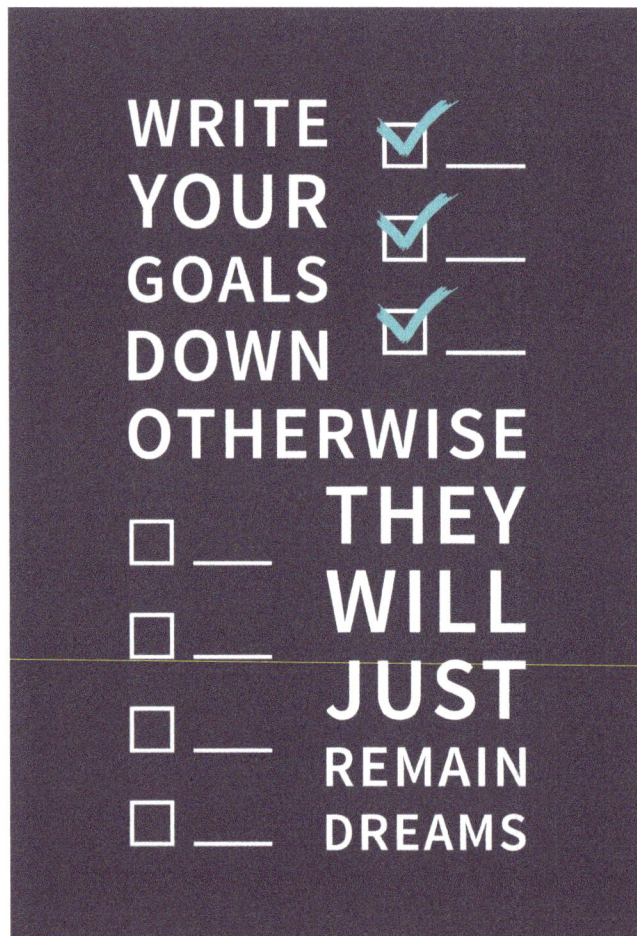

Do these exercises this week or in the near future.

1. Ask yourself what it is you want. Deep down, what is it that you desire in life? Write down your short-term goals. Think about where you want to be in three months, six months, a year, five years. Be as specific as possible. Use these as your guide. Write down your long-term goals. Think about where you want to be in ten years, 15 years, and 25 years. Writing these goals down makes them more concrete.

2. Set up a journal or a portion of your journal to evaluate your progress in a way that will be meaningful to you. When you look back a month from now, what will have made you feel that you are making real strides toward your increased well-being? For example, if you want to get fit, what will you use as a measure? How many times you worked out? How many times you ate healthy meals? How many pounds you lost? It should be a measure that matters to you.

3. Being able to visualise your goals will strengthen them in your mind and emotions. Find a whiteboard or corkboard (or anything that will work as a vision board). Go through magazines, tearing out anything you see that reminds you of your goals and dreams. Find an old stack of magazines and start going through them page by page. A spa weekend? Cut that picture out. A cooking course? Put a picture of a chef on the board. Use any pictures that will make your goals and dreams real for you.

4. We've talked about the power of an open heart. As time goes on and you feel frustrated by some of the things that happen in your life, one thing that will keep you strong and positive is practising gratitude. Be thankful. Spend a few moments each day remembering and saying aloud what you are thankful for—material things, acts of kindness, your own peace and contentment, or other people. Whatever it is, be grateful for it. It can improve your mood immediately.

5. Practise mindfulness especially diligently when you feel that something is bothering you. Examine what's going on in your life at the moment and look at your thoughts and beliefs. Are certain thoughts getting in the way of your increased well-being? Could they cause you to turn from achieving the things you want for yourself? Face them and deal with them. This is a technique you might want to enlist a few times each week.

## CONCLUSION

Five Ways to Well-being is about you finding your best life, starting now. Even though it's centred on you, it's not "self-centered" with the negative connotation that word has. In fact, it's just the opposite. Choosing to live your life on automatic pilot cheats not just you, but your friends, family, community, and even the world of experiencing you at your best.

The greatest power you have is your ability to choose the way you perceive life and the choices you make about how you will act. It's a responsibility, but also a great gift. Here's a brief reminder of the steps in the program and why they are important to you:

### Connect

Study after study has shown that the happiest people have the largest network of friends, colleagues, acquaintances, etc. It may go back to the "open heart" idea. When you are open to others, it doesn't just make them happier, it makes you happier. We all have so many ways to meet people. Even a smile and a "Hi" can brighten the day for both of you. Social networks on the internet can be a good place to make friends but get out there in the world to make some human contact, too.

## Be Active

This is not news to any of us—exercise makes us happy. Okay, for some of us, we're not very happy when we're actually doing it, but even 20 or 30 minutes can raise your serotonin, phenylethylamine and endorphin levels, the natural chemicals that make you feel good. You don't even have to go to the gym. Just walk for 30 minutes a few days a week to enjoy a great happiness boost. You'll boost the oxygen level in your brain and increase your focus and short-term memory at the same time. You might even start to see a trimmer body, which is a step toward increased well-being.

## Take Notice

Many people are afraid to take too close a look at themselves because they might not be as good as they hope and even worse than they suspect. That sizes up our fears perhaps, but it's just negative mental chatter, not reality. As you continue to practise mindfulness, you will get better at thinking clear, good-feeling thoughts. Better thoughts lead to better actions, which lead to better results. You are always just one mindful minute away from controlling your negative thoughts and feelings by understanding them and replacing them with less dysfunctional, more positive ones. Also, the world is full of rewarding experiences that will pass you by unless you trade your automatic living for mindfulness.

## Keep Learning

Did you know that studies have shown that there are two types of mindsets: fixed mindsets and growth mindsets? It's true. A person with a fixed mindset believes that his abilities are fixed and that he has a certain amount of talent and that's it. He avoids challenges so he won't have to risk failing. He plays it safe so he won't get any criticism or negative feedback. A person with a growth mindset believes that his intelligence and abilities can be trained. He embraces challenges because he sees them as opportunities to improve himself and develop new skills. His self-image is not tied to his successes, and he sees failure and negative feedback as an opportunity to learn. He feels good about how much effort he puts in, not whether he succeeds or fails. His goal is to improve.

Which type of person will have the more interesting life?

## Give

We were taught it as children, and now the science proves it to be true—it's good to give. It helps the other person, and it helps you. It doesn't have to be fancy or expensive. Take chocolate into work for sharing, even when it's not a special occasion. Thank your boss for her support. Plant a tree. Put your shopping cart back in the rack. Be nice to someone who looks lonely. Smile! Volunteer at a nearby shelter. Big things, small things— just give. Your attitude might be a bigger gift than the gift itself.

## The Critical ½ Step

Since Five Ways to Well-being is about you increasing your well-being by doing things you want to do, chose to sign up for, and are committed to, your motivation should be fairly steady. If you are involved in something you don't like doing at all, you should practise some mindful thinking about it to find out if there's a way to change the situation for the better. From time to time, though, you may not feel like following through on things you signed up for. This five-minute technique can be a great motivator for you. If there's something you just don't want to do (exercise, clean the garage), do it for just five minutes. You'll be surprised that the time went by so fast, and it wasn't as painful as you thought it would be. The next day, you'll feel better about the main task.

Your life may be okay, maybe even easy in some ways if you operate on automatic pilot and choose not to practise Five Ways to Well-being. But it won't be as interesting, rewarding, or satisfying on the deepest level. My promise to you is that your journey to well-being will be the most exciting one you have ever taken, full of fulfilling experiences you haven't envisioned yet.

> *"You've got a life to live. It's short, at best. It's a wonderful privilege and a terrific opportunity — and you've been equipped for it. Use your equipment. Give it all you've got. Love your neighbour — he's having just as much trouble as you are. Be nice to him; be kind to him. Trust God. And work hard."*
> —Norman Vincent Peale

# NUTRITION FOR WELL-BEING

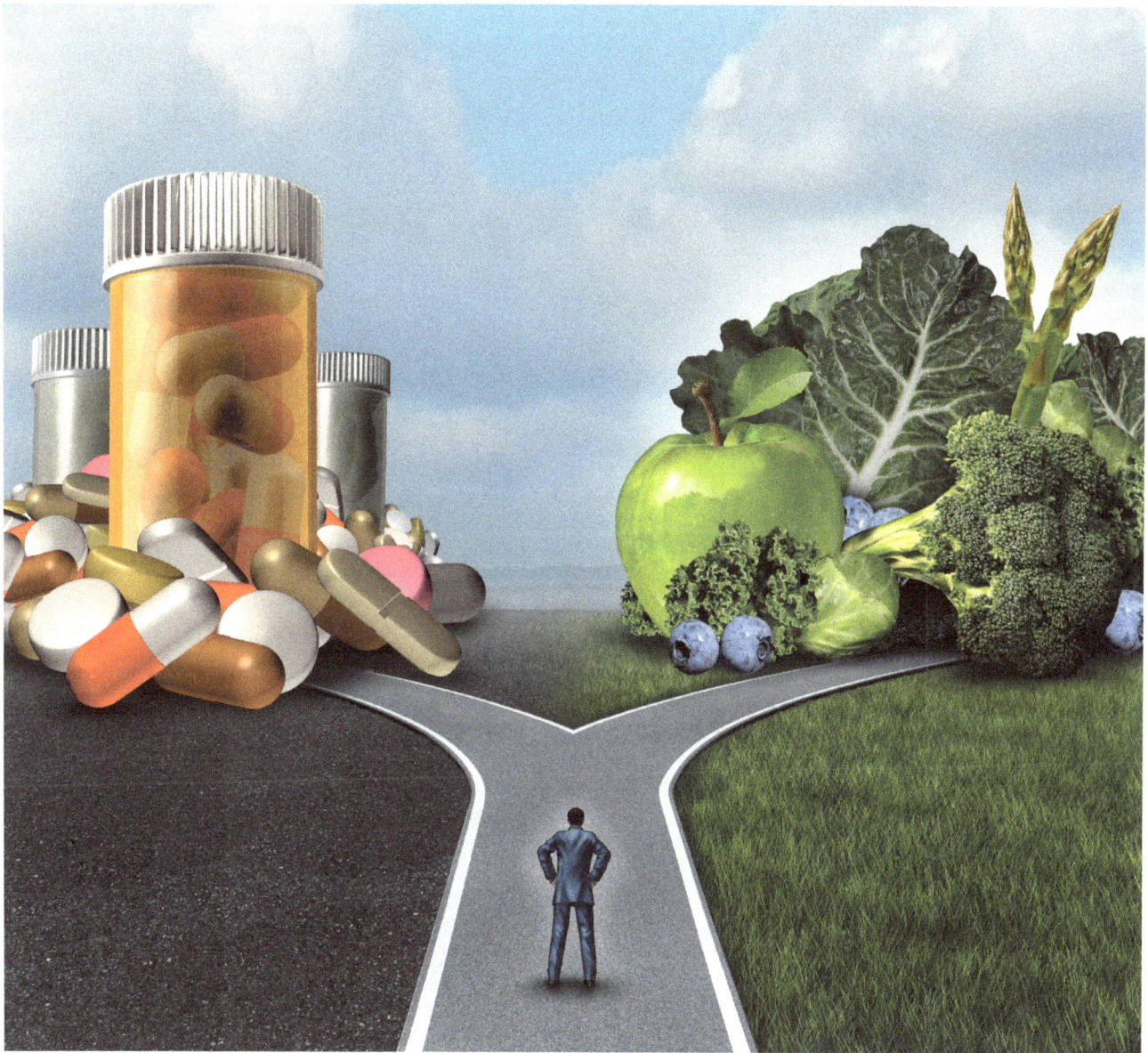

The Foresight Project (FP) which communicated the evidence base for improving people's well-being acknowledges that a balanced diet is important for well-being. This is further reinforced by The National Institute for Mental Health in England that highlights 'eating well' in its framework for improving mental health and well-being in England.

However, according to the Foresight Project, they did not include an action on the theme of nutrition for three reasons.

1. FP argues that the evidence on the role of different nutritional factors is complex so that the direct links between eating well and feeling good remain ambiguous until more research is completed.

My response: I totally agree that research around nutrition is very confusing and I believe we need to go with the best evidence we have at hand today as nutrition is very important. This bonus chapter will aim to remove the wheat from the chaff so that you are clearer what to eat for well-being.

2. FP's aim was to choose the most accessible interventions. Therefore, FP choices were, to some extent, dictated by those activities that were not reliant on external resources (like money, access to retail outlets, etc.) for their user-friendly appeal.

My response: I totally respect this as the nutritional world is very commercial and a lot of lobbying/marketing is done by the food industry to sell the food to the public as healthy food. It is of great benefit to have focused on the five ways to well-being, but nutrition is medicine and is the key to health. Hippocrates illustrated this by this famous phrase" Let thy food be thy medicine."

3. FP mentions that "the UK population has been messaged on healthy eating for the promotion of physical health, so FP felt there was less of a priority to raise awareness on this theme."

My response: I do not agree with this statement. If the UK population has been messaged properly on healthy eating why according to the Organisation for Economic Co-operation and Development (OECD) obesity rates have doubled over the past two decades in the UK. In fact, 63% of UK adults are overweight, and the UK one of the most obese nations in western Europe. There is clearly a priority to raise more awareness to the public about nutrition.

As I am not a nutritionist by trade, it took me over five years to write this chapter. I was not only reading books, attending workshops but also attended courses worth thousands of pounds by some of the top experts in the nutritional world. The more I learnt, the more confused I became because everybody was contradicting each other in the nutrition industry. They were even suing each other in the court of law. Although nutrition guidelines are supposed to help people eat healthily, they can have a very negative effect on consumers: they give nutritionists a bad name, they can be very confusing, and they decrease people's determination to follow the official nutrition recommendations.

More and more people are fed up with complicated nutritional advice, contradictory research studies, and endless health diets. According to research published in the Journal of Health Communication in 2014, most people find all this exhausting and confusing and, unfortunately, many are beginning to doubt the validity of even simple advice, such as "eat more fruit and veggies".

The two main reasons for this are:

1. The vast majority of research in nutrition is reductionist in nature. So far, the study of nutrition focused on one chemical at a time, in an attempt to determine its particular impact on the human body. These studies

helped food companies prove that processed foods did contain nutrition that is good for us. In *The China Study*, T. Colin Campbell provides the evidence that a whole food, plant-based diet is the healthiest way to eat. In his book *Whole*, he explains the ways our current scientific knowledge ignores the fascinating complexity of the human body.

The key issue he addresses in this book is why, if we have such overwhelming evidence that everything we think we know about nutrition is wrong, our eating habits haven't changed. The complexity of human body, as well as of the food itself, is forcing us to rethink everything we think we know about nutrition and healthy eating habits.

The vast majority of research in nutrition is reductionist in nature. As a reductionist, one believes that everything in the world can be understood if you understand its component parts. On the other hand, a holistic researcher emphasises the whole, rather than its constituent parts

2. Secondly, we need to embrace the concept of bio-individuality. We cannot fit everyone in one box and tell them what to eat. Hence, we could use models like the Food Pyramid, MyPlate, the UK Eatwell plate, are all unique and have specific nutrition needs depending on our age, constitution, gender, environment, lifestyle, blood types and ancestry. Bio-individuality teaches us to tune in to our own bodies and work out what sort of food, or lifestyle, suits us most. Forcing yourself to live a certain way or eat certain foods just because "everyone else does" is putting unnecessary pressure on your body (and mind) and is bound to fail. This is particularly true in the light of the globalisation and the loss of cultural diversity. As the world is becoming rapidly Westernised, the diets forced upon us through aggressive marketing campaigns are often very unhealthy. Adopting the diet that suits your particular needs is the best way to ensure long-term health and happiness. It takes maturity to ignore the pressure of being "in," i.e. to look or eat a certain way. Nor is it a guarantee that you will lose as much weight as someone else who follows the same diet.

But eventually, after coaching a lot of clients, I received my moment of epiphany. To explain my healthy eating concept and make it more palatable, I have devised a model called "the alchemist wellness plate". The alchemist wellness plate is a new paradigm shift in how we should view nutrition. Discovering the alchemist wellness plate is a blueprint for finding out what food works for you and how best to incorporate it into your diet. Rather than experimenting with food hypes and nutritional supplements, go for simple, wholesome and health-promoting foods that have stood the test of time.

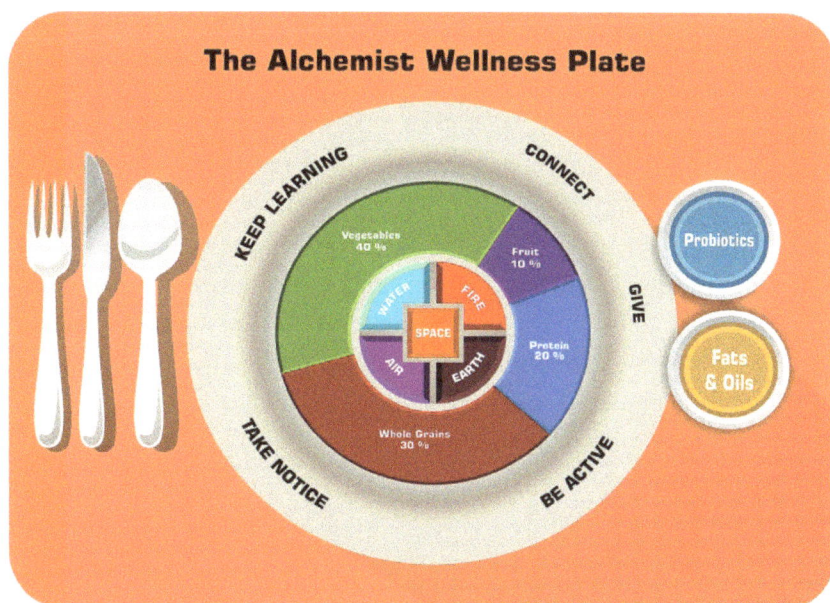

**The Alchemist Wellness Plate**

There are six areas of the alchemist wellness plate I want to discuss to complete my discussion about nutrition for well-being:

1. The spoon, fork and knife.
2. Probiotics
3. Fats and oils
4. The inner plate (Five elements: water, fire, air, water, fire, space)
5. The mid-plate (vegetables: eat the rainbow), fruits, protein and whole grains)
6. The outer plate (connect: be active, give, connect. keep learning)

## The Spoon fork and knife.

This is a metaphor for the mechanics of eating. This is about how you eat. The big ongoing debate in the nutrition industry is about what should we be eating. What is healthy and what is not healthy?

All good experts in the nutrition industry will tell you actually how and when you eat is more important what you eat. Let me repeat this: How, why and when we eat is more important than what we eat. Then, I am sure you'll be questioning me and asking me why our well-being is dictated by "we are what we eat." To this, I would answer: Nutrition for well-being is based on what our bodies digest and also what we successfully eliminate. The spoon, fork and knife metaphor, for me, is that we need to be conscious of our eating. Chew each mouthful of food 10-20 times. This is crucial as digestion starts in the mouth. We must chew our food properly and savour it like a gourmet meal and enjoy the texture, smell and flavours of each mouthful. Do not forget to you're your fork after every mouthful and pick it up again after every ten seconds or so. The adventure of eating for well-being only starts with conscious eating.

## Why do we eat?

Human beings eat mainly for the following six reasons:

1. To regulate and maintain our bodily functions
2. To get energy so that this uplifts our mood
3. To help us create a strong immune system that helps prevent and fight disease
4. To help us have a good physical appearance
5. To cleanse the body and get rid of toxins
6. For social situations and enjoyment

There is nothing wrong if the reasons we eat are those listed above. However, the golden rule is that we should only be eating when we are hungry.

Another key reason that I conveniently forgot to mention above is emotional eating. Emotional eating is comfort eating to help us to numb our real emotions, and it has nothing to do with physical hunger, so that's why many people think they never feel full—they never get the signal to stop eating because they were never hungry for food in the first place. Real hunger is a simple physical feeling in your stomach that builds gradually, which is worth waiting for and it's not the feeling you get when you walk past your favourite bakery or restaurant.

Emotional eating causes overeating has been officially classified by World Health Organisation as an eating disorder, and more than 2.5 million in the UK suffer from it. Emotional eating needs to be tackled if we are to eat healthily.

Please see some tips below about how and when we eat:

1. Eat consciously and get rid of any distractions like TV, smartphones. Make eating a ritual and focus on your eating. More importantly, enjoy every mouthful
2. Sit comfortably
    Whenever possible, try to eat at a table, sitting in a comfortable chair and being relaxed as much as possible. If you're feeling tense or anxious, you'll do yourself a favour by refraining from food.
3. Chew well and eat slowly
    Chewing thoroughly is good for digestion, as the food is already half-digested by the time it reaches the stomach. Eating slowly makes you eat mindfully.
4. Refrain from liquid
    Take as little liquid during the meal as possible (one small teacup of herbal tea or warm water if you have to). Water should be taken 30 minutes before, and two hours after the meal as they tend to dilute the digestive juices
5. Do not eat foods or drink ice-cold beverages
    Fire needed to help digest food eventually gets dampened and weak, possibly even extinguished, if you continually eat food straight from the fridge, or "cooling" foods such as raw salads and cold drinks.
6. Know when to stop
    Stop before you start feeling full. The overloaded stomach makes you feel tired, lazy and congested. It's very unhealthy and may lead to obesity.

## 2. Probiotics

Your gut health shows how healthy, or unhealthy you are. Today, digestive problems are becoming so common that they threaten to turn into an epidemic, and they can start even in early childhood. The number of prescribed drugs and over-the-counter drugs for digestive disorders like Maalox and Tagamet have soared considerably through the years, and this is a testament to our poor gut health in general.

While for the most common ones, such as irritable bowel syndrome, celiac disease, reflux, constipation and food intolerances, a lifestyle change often helps. However, in the case of chronic problems, you may have to boost your digestive powers with pro- and prebiotics.

In the post-antibiotic world, when we are trying to understand all of the consequences of the antibiotic overuse and misuse, we finally realised that for our gut to work, we have to continually feed it good bacteria and other microorganisms to keep it working smoothly.

However, it's not just the overuse of antibiotics that has undermined our gut flora and immune system. It is the overuse of pesticides, insecticides, growth hormones in animal feed, and all the other chemical pollutants we so carelessly use to "protect" ourselves from bacteria and pests. This irresponsible overuse of chemicals increased our toxicity to such levels that despite much higher living standards than 100 years ago, our global health is deteriorating fast.

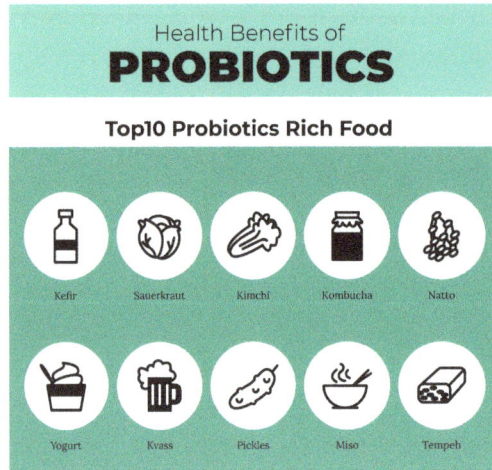

For our intestinal flora to stay healthy, we need a diet rich in probiotics.

Probiotics work in different ways:

➤ Probiotics are live bacteria which can be taken in the natural form, e.g. in yoghurt or sauerkraut, but it is also available as a tablet.
➤ They offer relief for most digestive troubles, for they add live bacteria which boosts digestion.
➤ Probiotics keep harmful bacteria in balance
➤ They aid digestion and nutrient absorption
➤ They contribute to a healthy immune system

## 3. Fats and Oils

Our body needs fat for energy, to absorb vitamins, and to ensure healthy heart and brain function. There are "good" and "bad" fats. "Bad" fats, such as artificial trans fats and saturated fats, contribute towards weight gain, clogged arteries, etc.

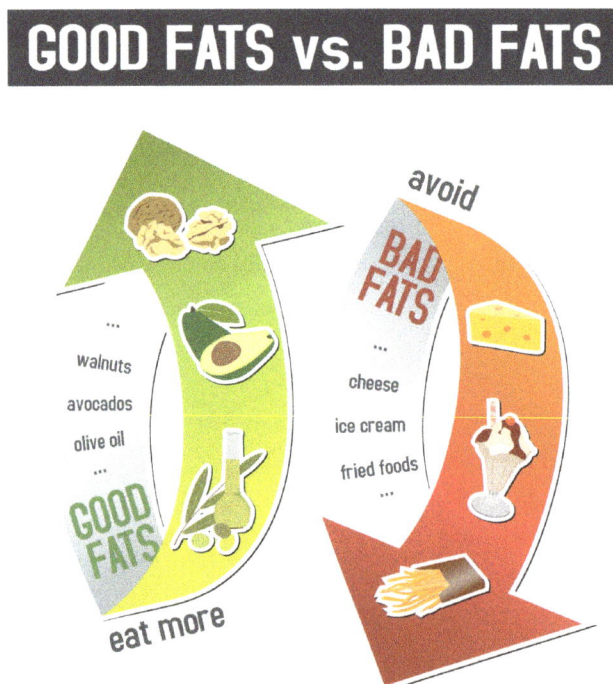

On the other hand, the "good" fats, such as unsaturated fats and omega-3s, help us manage our moods, fight fatigue, and can even help with weight loss.

To access the appropriate amounts of healthy fats, I recommend fats from whole food sources, such as nuts, seeds, avocados and olives, which contain a whole host of other nutrients that are beneficial to your body.

For health reasons, I would not recommend that you use any processed oils like sunflower oil, rapeseed oil. And this also includes limiting fried foods to a minimum.

**4. The inner plate is a reminder to us that nutrition for well-being is what gives us energy.
The inner plate is what traditionally in the East and now backed by scientific research in
the west about the importance of the five elements (Fire, air, water, space, earth).**

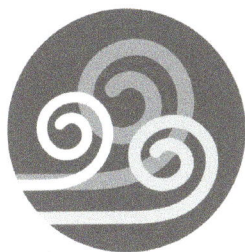
Air

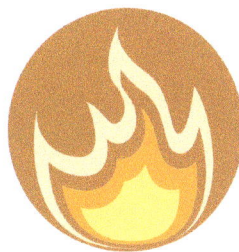
Fire

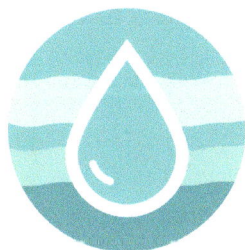
Water

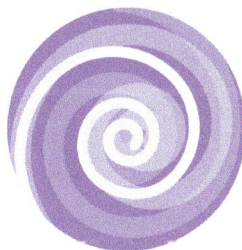
Ether

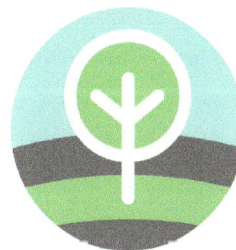
Earth

The five elements that provide the foundation for well-being

– Air element

The importance of oxygen for all life on Earth is self-explanatory. All living beings (plants, animals and humans) need air to breathe, and without it, there would be no life on Earth.

Today, many scientists believe that most of us suffer from a lack of oxygen. This may be because of improper breathing, poor diet, air pollution or lack of exercise. Whatever the reason for this may be, our cells are being deprived of this vital life-supporting element, and this deficiency is also weakening our immune system. Remember, the number one nutrient for our cells is oxygen!

– Water element

About 60-70% of the human body is made up of water, although this varies with age, gender, weight and body composition. Most of this water is in the organs, e.g. the brain is 85% water and about 90% of the blood flowing through your veins is also water. This explains why adequate hydration is so important for our health. Every cell, tissue, and organ in your body needs water to work properly because the body uses water to maintain its temperature, remove waste, and lubricate your joints.

– Space/ether element

Space is all around us. When the space element is balanced, you are able to freely communicate, express yourself, feel connected to the world around you, and feel physically and emotionally nourished. An unbalanced space element may lead you to feel empty, isolated, overwhelmed, withdrawn, and misunderstood. In Ayurvedic medicine, the element space is described as ethereal and spiritual and is connected with conscious awareness. Space for me is spiritual nourishment for the soul. Are you doing enough to feed your soul?

– Fire element

As the main source of "fire", the Sun has always stood for life, light, warmth and ultimately, happiness. But, it also has many health benefits. Exposure to the ultraviolet radiation causes your skin to create vitamin D. On the other hand, there is evidence that a moderate amount of sunlight actually has a cancer preventative benefit. Sun also helps relieve many skin conditions. Spending time in the open is also very beneficial for mental health. Exposure to sunlight releases a hormone serotonin, the so-called "feel good" hormone, which is triggered by sunlight that goes through the eye. Therefore, it'll do you good to spend some time in the Sun without sunglasses.

– Earth element

Clay has been used for thousands of years, both internally, and externally. Internally, it helps with digestion, enhances tissue repair, absorbs toxins and heavy metals, stimulates the immune system, reduces tension. It also helps you get rid of food poisons. Externally, you can apply it to your face as a beauty mask, or all over your body in wellness spas as a way of putting minerals into the body. It will clean and exfoliate the skin, clearing impurities and allergic reactions. All over Africa, it is still used as a face decoration during traditional festivals.

The element of earth is also used for its "grounding" benefits. Walking barefoot may sound crazy to many, but we walked and ran barefoot for over two million years. In many warm climate countries, people still do. And like everything else that increases your contact with nature, walking barefoot boosts your health in so many ways—it improves both your balance and your circulation, it boosts your mood, and by stimulating nerves on the soles of your feet, it helps reduce inflammation, pain and tension.

## 5. The mid-plate is:

Basically, the mid-plate is food that we eat. Our diets vary, but they usually revolve around a different combination of

1. Vegetables (40%)
2. Whole grains (30%)
3. Proteins (20%)
4. Fruits (10%)

The above should be the building blocks of our diet.

- Vegetables

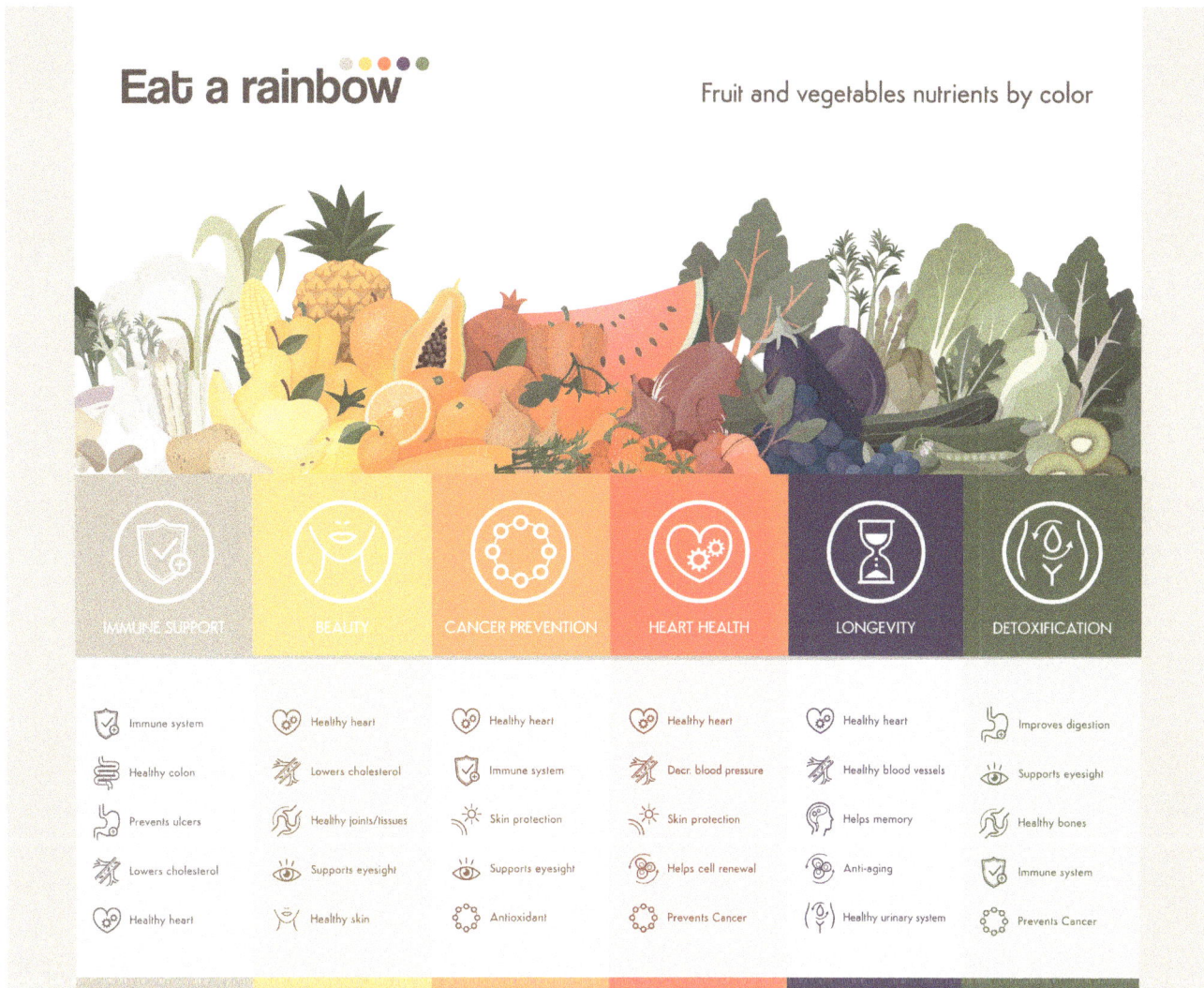

When it comes to veggies, it is not a surprise that it accounts for 40 percent of what we should be eating as part of a healthy diet because they are loaded with powerful nutrients. When we talk about eating vegetables, it's best to eat a rainbow of colours. [118] That's because the colour of a vegetable is an indicator of the phytonutrients it contains. The more colours you eat, the larger the variety of nutrients you get.

Vegetables fall broadly into five different colour categories: red, purple/blue, orange, green and white/brown. Each colour carries its own set of unique disease-fighting chemicals called phytochemicals that give vegetables their healthy properties.

Let's look at the colours:

RED

Red vegetables contain the following nutrients: lycopene, ellagic acid, quercetin, and hesperidin. These nutrients reduce the risk of cancer, lower blood pressure, and LDL cholesterol levels, and scavenge harmful free-radicals. E.g. red peppers, tomatoes, radish.

## PURPLE /BLUE

The plant pigment anthocyanin is what gives blue/purple vegetables their distinctive colour. Anthocyanin also has antioxidant properties that protect cells from damage and can help boost immune system activity, support healthy digestion, improve calcium and other mineral absorption and fight inflammation. E.g. eggplant. Purple cabbage, purple asparagus.

## ORANGE/YELLOW

Carotenoids give this group their vibrant colour. A well-known carotenoid called beta-carotene is found in sweet potatoes, pumpkins and carrots. It is converted to vitamin A, which helps maintain healthy mucous membranes and healthy eyes. Another carotenoid called lutein is stored in the eye and has been found to prevent cataracts and age-related macular degeneration, which can lead to blindness.

## GREEN

Green foods contain chemicals that help ward off cancer by inhibiting carcinogens. Chlorophyll is the component that makes plants green and is purifying in the body. Many green foods also contain calcium and minerals.

Green foods include

- Kale, spinach and other leafy greens
- Green apples
- Artichokes
- Sea vegetables

## BROWN/WHITE

Nutrients in white fruits and vegetables include beta-glucans and lignans that provide powerful immune boosting activity. These nutrients also activate natural killer B and T cells, reduce the risk of cancers and balance hormone levels, reducing the risk of hormone-related cancers.

Brown/ white veggies include cauliflower, dates, ginger, jerusalem artichoke, kohlrabi.

**Action**: If you struggle to eat a lot of vegetables, a creative way to ensure we have a good variety of vegetables in our diet is via juicing vegetables or vegetable smoothies. If you do not have a blender or juicer, please buy one. If money is an issue,Jack Lallane who is known as the grandfather of fitness used to say " If you do not have a juicer, sell your car and buy one. It will take you further in life than your car". Joking aside, this will be one of the best investment you will do in terms of your well being. As far as blenders are concerned, there are some popular brand on the market that I recommend like Nutribullet or Vitamix if you want to go high end.

- Whole Grains

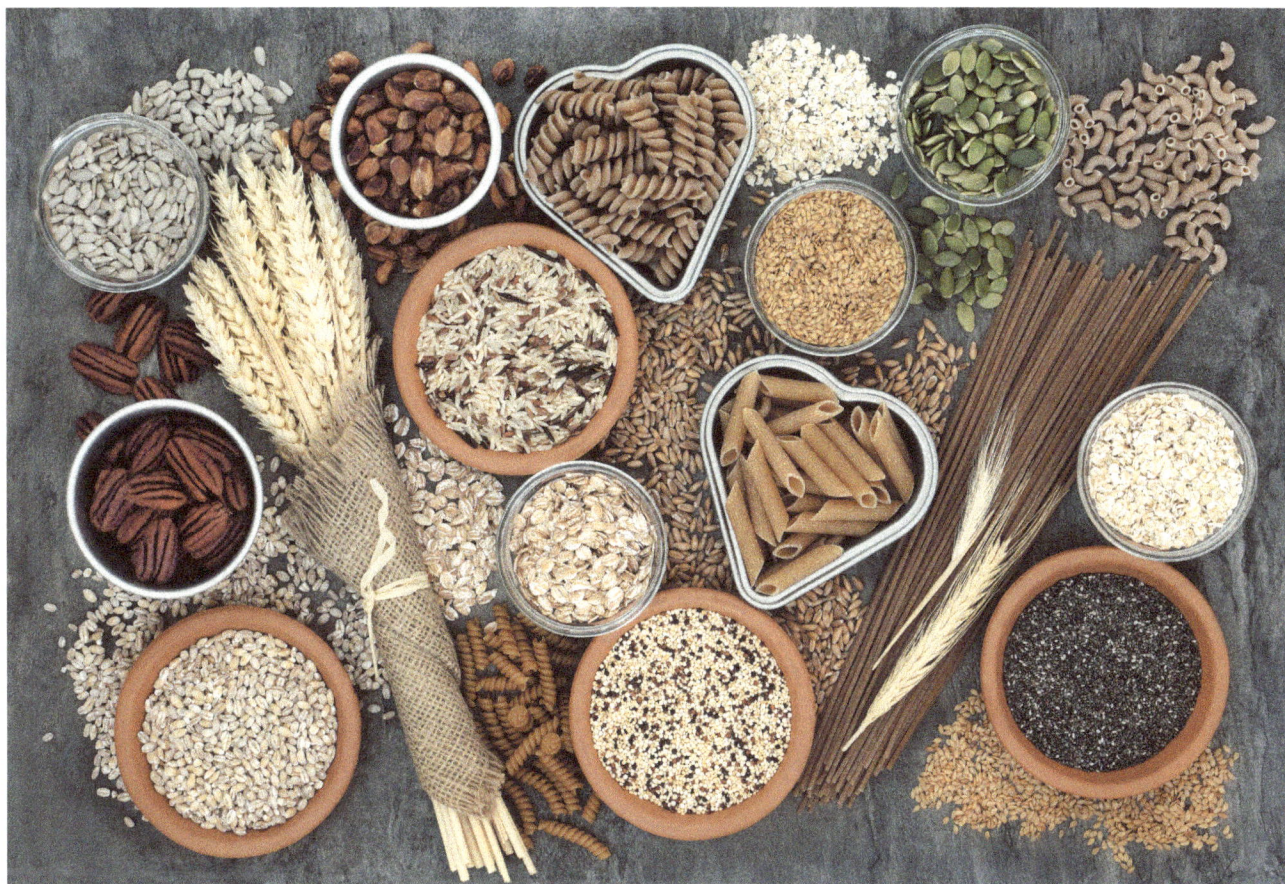

Whole grains have been demonised by the media as we live in the era of low carb. The fact of the matter is whole grains are health-promoting.

What are whole grains in the first place?

According to Dr Stanger, "Whole grains are the seeds of certain grasses that store their energy mostly as complex carbohydrates. Wheat, corn, rice, barley, oats, millet, and rye are the most common examples. Whole grain foods contain all parts of the seed: the outer protective skin (bran), the tiny baby plant (the germ), and food to nourish the baby plant until it can produce its own (endosperm)." [119]

I would also include quinoa, buckwheat, wild rice, and amaranth to the family of whole grains although they are produced by plants.

Peer-reviewed studies show that there are lots of health benefits to individuals who consume healthy foods. Here are three key ones:

1.  Whole Grains Reduce Your Risk of Obesity
    In the field of nutrition, a myth that needs to be demystified is that foods high in carbohydrates cause obesity. However, peer-reviewed research finds quite the opposite. An example is an analysis of fifteen research trials with data from 119,829 participants concluded that a higher intake of whole grains was linked to lower BMI and waist size.

2.  Whole Grains Decrease Your Risk of Chronic Illness

People who consume whole grains have less chance of developing the chronic degenerative illnesses. Moreover, eating more whole grains is linked to lower levels of a common inflammatory marker associated with chronic disease.

3.  Whole Grains Help You Live Longer

In 2015, researchers published an analysis of two large studies of participants followed for approximately 25 years. They reported that each additional one-ounce daily serving of whole grains reduced the risk of death over the study period by 5%, and the risk of death from cardiovascular disease by 9%. The beneficial effect was seen from the combined effects of many foods, including whole wheat and whole-wheat flour, oats, corn and popcorn, rye, brown rice, and whole-grain breakfast cereals.

Researchers and nutritionists cite a number of reasons that whole grains could have a positive effect on health. Whole grains high fibre content makes food more satisfying, and whole grains promote beneficial gut microbes, which produce protective short-chain fatty acids. Wholegrains are also dense with vitamins, minerals, amino acids, antioxidants, and phytochemicals.

*   Protein

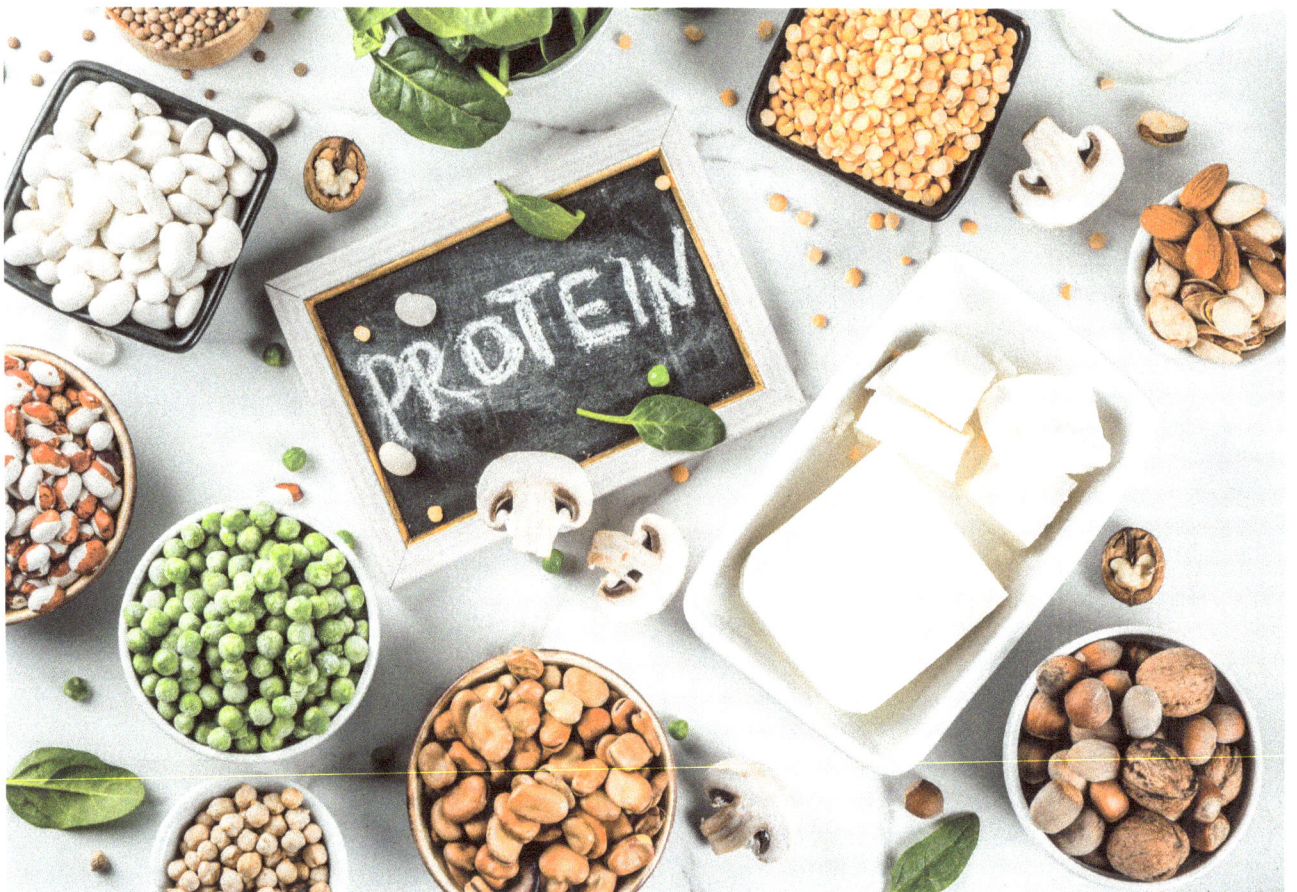

Protein represents the building block of our cells, tissues and organs. There are 20 different amino acids needed by the body. These amino acids join together to make all different types of protein. The average recommended intake of protein is 42 grams a day. Non-vegetarians eat way more than that (almost 80 grams), but so does everyone else. Vegetarians and vegans actually average 70% more protein than they need every day (over 70 grams). There is so much fuss over protein when, actually, we are all taking excess proteins. I highly recommend taking proteins from plant-based sources, e.g. black, kidney, pinto, and other beans, almonds, lentils, hemp seeds, spirulina, and quinoa.

- Fruits

The nutrients in fruits are vital for health and maintenance of your body. It's essential to eat a variety of types and colours in order to give your body the mix of nutrients it needs. With fruits, it is important not to overindulge as fruits can have much sugar in them. Fruits, as delicious as they can be, contain fructose. And fructose is a problem because it can ONLY be metabolised by the liver. We were not designed to eat the vast volumes of fructose we now eat. I would eat mainly alkaline fruits, like below, and minimise eating sweet fruit that can be very acidic. As a rule, 80 percent of our diet should be alkaline and 20 percent acidic. For most people the reverse is true.

Alkaline Fruits List

- Lemon
- Lime
- Avocado
- Cucumber
- Tomato
- Grapefruit
- Pomegranate

# ACID / ALKALINE FOOD
## COMPARISON CHART

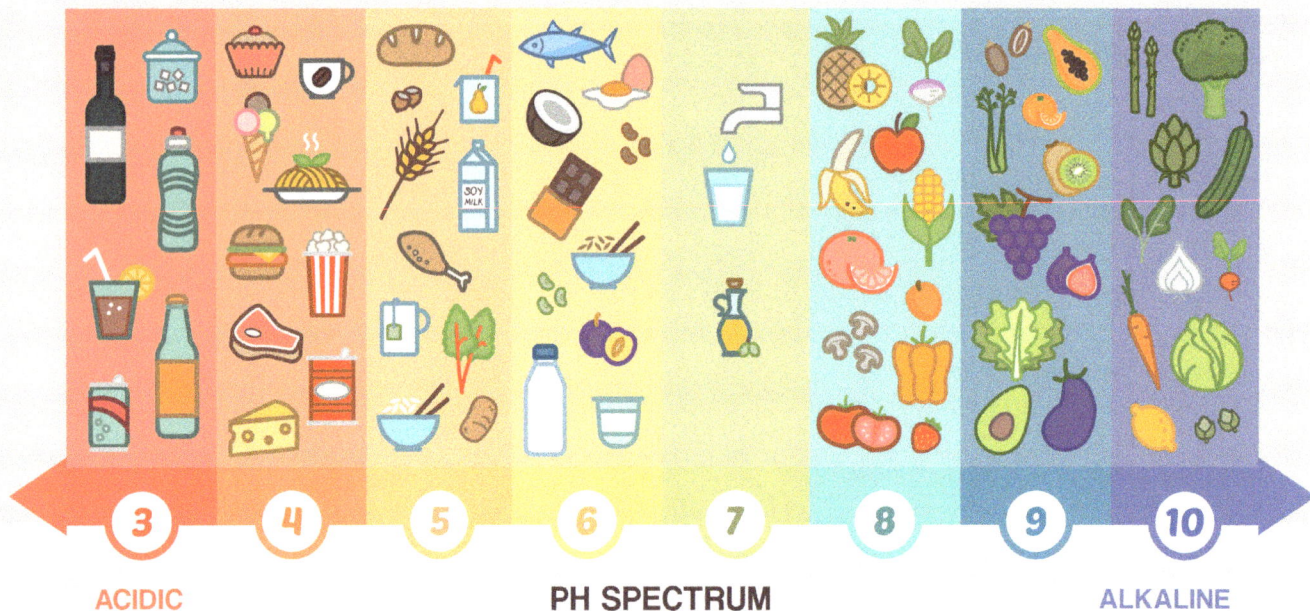

**3** **4** **5** **6** **7** **8** **9** **10**

**ACIDIC**        **PH SPECTRUM**        **ALKALINE**

## THE ACID / ALKALINE
### BALANCED DIET

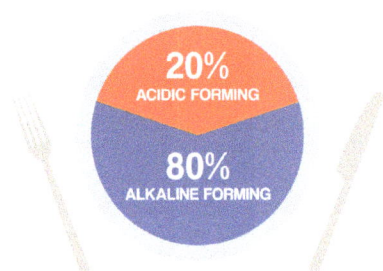

20% ACIDIC FORMING

80% ALKALINE FORMING

### THE 7 MOST ALKALINE FOODS

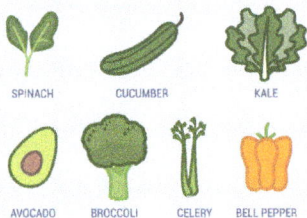

SPINACH    CUCUMBER    KALE

AVOCADO    BROCCOLI    CELERY    BELL PEPPER

## HEALTH BENEFITS
### ON YOUR BODY

IMPROVES MEMORY AND COGNITION

PROMOTES CARDIOVASCULAR HEALTH

BOOST IMMUNE SYSTEM

BETTER DIGESTION

PREVENTS CANCER

KEEPS BONES AND MUSCLES HEALTHY

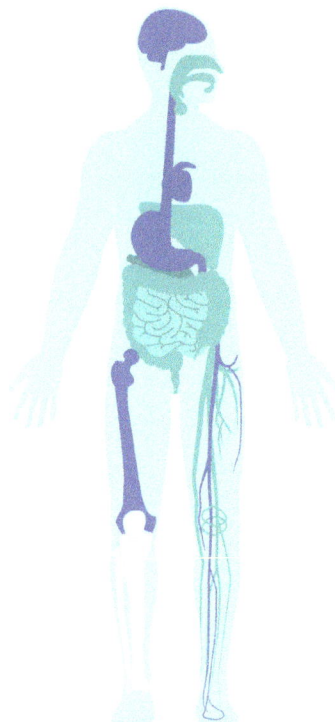

## 6. The outer plate

The outer plate is to emphasise the importance of the five ways to well-being in nutrition which we have covered extensively in this book. We've discussed how connecting can be nourishing in chapter 1. Being active is a requisite for healthy eating, not only to burn calories but also to stimulate the lymphatic system of the body so we can eliminate properly. Being aware is an important component of eating in terms of mindful eating to enhance our digestive process and hence our body's assimilation of food. Keeping up with learning is always useful as there is always new information in the nutrition world that we need to learn to stay ahead of the curve and not be a victim of cheap sales food marketing. Eventually "giving" is fascinating. Sharing our food with others will increase our well-being.

In a nutshell, in terms of nutrition for well-being, I would recommend you address all the areas of the alchemist wellness plate. In terms of food choices, based on my extensive research, I would recommend a whole foods plant-based diet and this is based on *The China Study* by T Colin Campbell, PhD. [120] This is considered the most comprehensive nutrition study ever conducted.

It revolves around the idea that a plant-based diet not only promotes good health, but has the power to prevent or reverse many diseases.

Moreover, Dr Campbell has summarised the 8,000 statistically significant correlations found in the China Study in the following statement: "people who ate whole foods, plant-based diet are more healthy."

Action:

1. Revisit the alchemist wellness plate on a daily basis and ensure that you are taking care of all the six areas of the plate so that you can have holistic nutrition
2. Remember I do not recommend a vegan or vegetarian lifestyle in terms of foods as those diets can be loaded with sugar and refined foods. I advocate for a whole foods, plant-based (WFPB) lifestyle
3. For more exposure on leading a whole foods, plant-based (WFPB) lifestyle, I strongly recommend the documentary movie Forks Over Knives, which is also available on Netflix. Forks Over Knives [121] is a documentary that advocates a low fat, whole foods plant-based diet as a way to avoid or reverse several chronic diseases. The film highlights that processed foods and all oils should be avoided. As the WFPB lifestyle would be new to many of you reading this book, I am sure you'll ask me about recipes. The Forks over Knives website has some brilliant recipes that I highly recommend. In consultation with your doctor, give the WFPB diet a go for at least 4 weeks and note any changes to your wellbeing.
4. Eventually, remember the concept of Bio-individuality. When it comes to nutrition, your body knows best, listen to it and learn from its wisdom.

# BIBLIOGRAPHY

1   Mendelsohn M. Positive Psychology: The Science of Happiness. [Internet] abcNEWS 2008 Jan. Available from: http://abcnews.go.com/Health/story?id=4115033

2   Mendelsohn M. Positive Psychology: The Science of Happiness. [Internet] abcNEWS 2008 Jan. Available from: http://abcnews.go.com/Health/story?id=4115033&page=3

3   Cameron D. PM Speech on Wellbeing. GOV>UK. [serial online]2010 Nov. Available from: https://www.gov.uk/government/speeches/pm-speech-on-wellbeing

4   Helliwell J, Layard R, Sachs J. The Happiest Countries Are in Northern Europe [serial online] 2012 Mar. Available from: http://www.huffingtonpost.com/john-helliwell/happiness-report_b_1391510.html

5   Hall Layard Sachs j. World Happiness Report [serial online] UN Conference on Sustainable Development 2012 Apr. Available from: http://issuu.com/earthinstitute/docs/world-happiness-report/10

6   Hall Layard Sachs J. World Happiness Report [serial online] UN Conference on Sustainable Development 2012 Apr. Available from: http://issuu.com/earthinstitute/docs/world-happiness-report/10

7   Foresight Programme, The Mental Capital and Wellbeing Project [serial online] 2008 Dec. Available from: http://www.bis.gov.uk/assets/foresight/docs/mental-capital/mentalcapitalwellbeingexecsum.pdf p.11.

8   Foresight Programme, The Mental Capital and Wellbeing Project [serial online] 2008 Dec. Available from: http://www.bis.gov.uk/assets/foresight/docs/mental-capital/final_project_report_part2.pdf p.11.

9   Foresight Programme, The Mental Capital and Wellbeing Project [serial online] 2008 Dec. Available from: http://www.bis.gov.uk/assets/foresight/docs/mental-capital/final_project_report_part2.pdf p.11.

10   Foresight Programme, The Mental Capital and Wellbeing Project [serial online] 2008 Dec. Available from: http://www.bis.gov.uk/assets/foresight/docs/mental-capital/final_project_report_part2.pdf p.18.

11   Foresight Programme, The Mental Capital and Wellbeing Project [serial online] 2008 Dec. Available from: http://www.bis.gov.uk/assets/foresight/docs/mental-capital/final_project_report_part2.pdf p.18.

12   Foresight Programme, The Mental Capital and Wellbeing Project [serial online] 2008 Dec. Available from: http://www.bis.gov.uk/assets/foresight/docs/mental-capital/final_project_report_part2.pdf p.19.

13   Foresight Programme, The Mental Capital and Wellbeing Project [serial online] 2008 Dec. Available from: http://www.bis.gov.uk/assets/foresight/docs/mental-capital/final_project_report_part2.pdf p.19.

14   Foresight Programme, The Mental Capital and Wellbeing Project [serial online] 2008 Dec. Available from: http://www.bis.gov.uk/assets/foresight/docs/mental-capital/final_project_report_part2.pdf p.18.

[15]  Aked J, Marks N, Cordon C, Thompson S. NEF measuring well-being: a guide for practitioners [serial online] 2012 Jul
Available from:
http://www.businessballs.com/freespecialresources/Five_Ways_to_Well-being-NEF.pdf p.5.

[16]  Pontin E, Schwannauer M, Tai S, Kinderman P. A UK validation of a general measure of subjective well-being: the modified BBC subjective well-being scale (BBC-SWB) [serial online] 2013 Nov
Available from: http://www.hqlo.com/content/pdf/1477-7525-11-150.pdf

[17]  Tennent R, Hiller L, Fishwick R, Platt P, Joseph S, Weich S, et al., Wellbeing self-assessment tool [serial online] 2007 Nov.
Available from:
http://www.nhs.uk/Tools/Documents/Wellbeing%20self-assessment.htm

[18]  Tennent R, Hiller L, Fishwick R, Platt P, Joseph S, Weich S, et al., Well-being self-assessment tool [serial online] 2007 Nov.
Available from:
http://www.nhs.uk/Tools/Documents/Wellbeing%20self-assessment.htm

[19]  Aked J, Marks N, Cordon C, Thompson S. NEF measuring well-being: a guide for practitioners [serial online] 2012 Jul.
Available from:
http://www.businessballs.com/freespecialresources/Five_Ways_to_Well-being-NEF.pdf p.5

[20]  Aked J, Marks N, Cordon C, Thompson S. NEF measuring well-being: a guide for practitioners [serial online] 2012 Jul.
Available from:
http://www.businessballs.com/freespecialresources/Five_Ways_to_Well-being-NEF.pdf p.5.

[21]  Aked J, Marks N, Cordon C, Thompson S. NEF measuring well-being: a guide for practitioners [serial online] 2012 Jul.
Available from:
http://www.businessballs.com/freespecialresources/Five_Ways_to_Well-being-NEF.pdf p.5.

[22]  Aked J, Marks N, Cordon C, Thompson S. NEF measuring well-being: a guide for practitioners [serial online] 2012 Jul.
Available from:
http://www.businessballs.com/freespecialresources/Five_Ways_to_Well-being-NEF.pdf p.6.

[23]  Aked J, Marks N, Cordon C, Thompson S. NEF measuring well-being: a guide for practitioners [serial online] 2012 Jul.
Available from:
http://www.businessballs.com/freespecialresources/Five_Ways_to_Well-being-NEF.pdf p.6.

[24]  Brown, B. *The Gifts of Imperfection: let go of who you think you're supposed to be and embrace who you are.* Center City: Hazelden; 2010. p. ix.

[25]  Brown, B. *The Gifts of Imperfection: let go of who you think you're supposed to be and embrace who you are.* Center City: Hazelden; 2010. p. x.

[26]  Brown, B. *The Gifts of Imperfection: let go of who you think you're supposed to be and embrace who you are.* Center City: Hazelden; 2010. p. x.

[27]  Brown, B. *The Gifts of Imperfection: let go of who you think you're supposed to be and embrace who you are.* Center City: Hazelden; 2010. p. xi.

[28]  Brown, B. *The Gifts of Imperfection: let go of who you think you're supposed to be and embrace who you are.* Center City: Hazelden; 2010. p. xi.

[29] Brown, B. *The Gifts of Imperfection: let go of who you think you're supposed to be and embrace who you are.* Center City: Hazelden; 2010. p. xiii.

[30] Brown, B. *The Gifts of Imperfection: let go of who you think you're supposed to be and embrace who you are.* Center City: Hazelden; 2010. p. xiii.

[31] Brown, B. *The Gifts of Imperfection: let go of who you think you're supposed to be and embrace who you are.* Center City: Hazelden; 2010. p. xiv.

[32] Kreitzer MJ. Why personal relationships are important. U of Minn [serial online] 2013 Aug.
Available from:
http://www.takingcharge.csh.umn.edu/enhance-your-wellbeing/relationships/why-personal-relationships-are-important

[33] Kreitzer MJ. Why personal relationships are important. U of Minn [serial online] 2013 Aug.
Available from:
http://www.takingcharge.csh.umn.edu/enhance-your-wellbeing/relationships/why-personal-relationships-are-important

[34] Lawson K. Work on communication for healthy relationships. U of Minn [serial online] 2013 Aug.
Available from:
http://www.takingcharge.csh.umn.edu/enhance-your-well-being/relationships/work-communication-healthy-relationships

[35] How do our social networks affect personal wellbeing? U of Minn [serial online] 2013 Sep.
Available from:
http://www.takingcharge.csh.umn.edu/enhance-your-well-being/community/how-do-our-social-networks-affect-personal-well-being

[36] How do our social networks affect personal wellbeing? U of Minn [serial online] 2013 Sep.
Available from:
http://www.takingcharge.csh.umn.edu/enhance-your-wellbeing/community/how-do-our-social networks-affect-personal-wellbeing

[36a] Project MATCH Research Group . Matching alcoholism treatment to client heterogeneity: Project MATCH three-year drinking outcomes. Alcoholism: Clinical and Experimental Research, 1998, 22: 6, 1300-1311.

[37] Brown, B. *The Gifts of Imperfection: let go of who you think you're supposed to be and embrace who you are.* Centre City: Hazelden; 2010 p. 20.

[38] Beattie A. Social media and its effects on our emotional well-being. Metro [serial online] 2013 Aug.
Available from: http://metro.co.uk/2013/08/15/social-media-and-its-effects-on-our-emotional-well-being-3924915/

[39] Beattie A. Social media and its effects on our emotional wellbeing. Metro [serial online] 2013 Aug.
Available from: http://metro.co.uk/2013/08/15/social-media-and-its-effects-on-our-emotional-well-being-3924915/

[40] Connect to the earth and feel better! Earthing [serial online] 2013.
Available from: http://www.earthing.com/category_s/1823.htm

[41] Edblad P. How to breathe properly – a (surprisingly important complete guide) Selfication [serial online] 2013 Aug.
Available from: www.selfication.com/how-to-breathe/

42    Matousek M. Is the way you breathe bad for your health? Oprah [serial online] 2013 Mar.
Available from:
www.oprah.com/spirit/deep-breathing-methods-how-breathing-reduces-stress

43    Batmanghelidj F. The wonders of water: amazing secrets of health and wellness. Watercure [serial online] 2004 Dec.
Available from:
http://www.watercure.com/wondersofwater.html

44    Harvey F. UK green spaces worth at least L30bn a year in health and welfare, report finds. Guardian [serial online] 2011 Jun.
Available from:
http://www.theguardian.com/environment/2011/jun/02/uk-green-spaces-value

45    Smedley T. What impact do seas, lakes and rivers have on people's health? Guardian [serial online] 2013 Mar. Available from: www.theguardian.com/impact-seas-lakes-rivers-peoples-health

46    Smedley T. What impact do seas, lakes and rivers have on people's health? Guardian [serial online] 2013 Mar. Available from: www.theguardian.com/impact-seas-lakes-rivers-peoples-health

47    Mercola J. Sunlight.Mercola: Benefits of sun exposure [serial online] 2012 Sep.
Available from:
http://www.mercola.com/Downloads/bonus/benefits-of-sun-exposure/report.aspx

48    Mercola J. Sunlight.Mercola: Benefits of sun exposure [serial online] 2012 Sep.
Available from:
http://www.mercola.com/Downloads/bonus/benefits-of-sun-exposure/report.aspx

49    Mercola J. Sunlight.Mercola: Benefits of sun exposure [serial online] 2012 Sep.
Available from:
http://www.mercola.com/Downloads/bonus/benefits-of-sun-exposure/report.aspx

50    Mercola J. Sunlight.Mercola: Benefits of sun exposure [serial online] 2012 Sep.
Available from:
http://www.mercola.com/Downloads/bonus/benefits-of-sun-exposure/report.aspx

51    Lee I, Shiroma E, Lobelo F, Puska P, Blair S, Katzmarzyk P. Effect of physical inactivity on major non-communicable diseases worldwide: an analysis of burden of disease and life expectancy Lancet 380 (9838)219-229. DOI:10.1016/S0140-6736(12)61031-9
Accessed in July 2018 from:
http://www.thelancet.com

52    Lee I, Shiroma E, Lobelo F, Puska P, Blair S, Katzmarzyk P. Effect of physical inactivity on major non-communicable diseases worldwide: an analysis of burden of disease and life expectancy Lancet 380 (9838)219-229. DOI:10.1016/S0140-6736(12)61031-9
Accessed in July 2018 from:
http://www.thelancet.com

53    Benefits of exercise. NHS [serial online] 2013 Nov.
Available from:
http://www.nhs.uk/Livewell/fitness/Pages/whybeactive.aspx

54    Get active your way. NHS [serial online] 2013 Nov.
      Available from:
      http://www.nhs.uk/livewell/fitness/pages/activelifestyle.aspx

55    Physical activity guidelines for adults. NHS [serial online] 2013 Nov.
      Available from:
      http://www.nhs.uk/livewell/fitness/pages/physical-activity-guidelines-for-adults.aspx

56    Get fit for free. NHS [serial online] 2013 Jan.
      Available from: http://www.nhs.uk/livewell/fitness/pages/free-fitness.aspx

57    Walking for health. NHS [serial online] 2012 Jun.
      Available from: http://www.nhs.uk/livewell/getting-started-guides/pages/getting-started-walking.aspx

58    Running tips for beginners. NHS [serial online] 2012 Jun.
      Available from: http://www.nhs.uk/livewell/getting-started-guides/pages/getting-started-running.aspx

58b   Upstate Medical University [serial online] 2014
      Available from: http://www.upstate.edu/health/wellness

59    Fitness training tips. NHS [serial online] 2013 Jul.
      Available from:
      http://www.nhs.uk/livewell/olympics/pages/trainingtips.aspx

60    Possibly the Perfect Exercise! Wtlossres [serial online] 2014.
      Available from:
      https://www.weightlossresources.co.uk/exercise/reviews/rebounding.htm

61    Walker M, Carter A. The Benefits of Rebound Exercise: 33 Ways the Body responds [serial online]
      Available from:
      http://rebound-air.com/best_rebounding_33_ways.htm

62    Ten ways to get fit. NHS [serial online] 2012 Mar.
      Available from:
      http://www.nhs.uk/livewell/teenboys/pages/fungettingfit.aspx

63    Fitness training tips. NHS [serial online] 2013 Jul.
      Available from:
      http://www.nhs.uk/Livewell/olympics/Pages/Trainingtips.aspx

64    Niven D. *The 100 Simple Secrets of Successful People*. New York: Harper Collins; 2002. p. 36.

65    Niven D. *The 100 Simple Secrets of Successful People*. New York: Harper Collins; 2002 p. 35-6.

66    Harper B. *Are you ready!* New York: Random House; 2008. p. 36-40

67    Harper B. *Are you ready!* New York: Random House; 2008 p. 36-40.

68    Ellsworth B. *Living in love with yourself*. Salt Lake City: Breakthrough Pub; 1988. p. 1-3.

69    Williams M, Penman D. *Mindfulness: an eight-week plan for finding peace in a frantic world* [monograph online] New York; Rodale 2011. loc 202.

70  Williams M, Penman D. *Mindfulness: an eight-week plan for finding peace in a frantic world* [monograph online] New York; Rodale 2011. loc. 476.

71  Williams M, Penman D. *Mindfulness: an eight-week plan for finding peace in a frantic world* [monograph online] New York; Rodale 2011. loc. 486.

72  Williams M, Penman D. *Mindfulness: an eight-week plan for finding peace in a frantic world* [monograph online] New York; Rodale 2011. loc. 533.

73  Williams M, Penman D. *Mindfulness: an eight-week plan for finding peace in a frantic world* [monograph online] New York; Rodale 2011. loc. 652.

74  Williams M, Penman D. *Mindfulness: an eight-week plan for finding peace in a frantic world* [monograph online] New York; Rodale 2011. loc. 227.

75  Williams M, Penman D. *Mindfulness: an eight-week plan for finding peace in a frantic world* [monograph online] New York; Rodale 2011. loc. 535.

76  Williams M, Penman D. *Mindfulness: an eight-week plan for finding peace in a frantic world* [monograph online] New York; Rodale 2011. loc. 126.

77  Williams M, Penman D. *Mindfulness: an eight-week plan for finding peace in a frantic world* [monograph online] New York; Rodale 2011. loc. 818.

78  A guide to yoga. NHS [serial online] 2013 Jul.
Available from:
http://www.nhs.uk/Livewell/fitness/Pages/yoga.aspx

79  A guide to tai chi. NHS [serial online] 2013 Aug.
Available from:
http://www.nhs.uk/Livewell/fitness/Pages/taichi.aspx

80  What is Heartmath. Heartmath [serial online] 2012
Available from:
http://www.earthhearthomeopathy.com/heartmath.html

80b  Institute of heartmath.www.heartmath.org [serial online] 2014

81  Mind is a frequent, but not happy, wanderer: people spend nearly half their waking hours thinking about what isn't going on around them. Harvard [serial online] 2012 Nov.
Available from:
http://www.sciencedaily.com/releases/2010/11/101111141759.htm

82  Mind is a frequent, but not happy, wanderer: people spend nearly half their waking hours thinking about what isn't going on around them. Harvard [serial online] 2012 Nov.
Available from:
http://www.sciencedaily.com/releases/2010/11/101111141759.htm

83  Grenville-Cleave B. *Positive Psychology: A Practical Guide.* [monograph online] Ontario: Icon; 2012. loc. 1687.

84  Grenville-Cleave B. *Positive Psychology: A Practical Guide.* [monograph online] Ontario: Icon; 2012. loc. 467.

85  How to feel happier. NHS [serial online] 2012 Dec.
Available from: http://www.nhs.uk/conditions/stress-anxiety-depression/pages/feel-better-and-happy.aspx

86  Diener E, Biswas-Diener R. *Happiness: unlocking the mysteries of psychology* [monograh online] Blackwell: Oxford; 2008. p. 244-5.

87  Diener E, Biswas-Diener R. *Happiness: unlocking the mysteries of psychology* [monograh online] Blackwell: Oxford; 2008. p. 244-5.

88  Christian K. *Your own worst enemy: breaking the habit of adult underachievement.* New York: Norton; 2002. p. 193-4.

89  Christian K. Your Own Worst Enemy: breaking the habit of adult underachievement. New York: Norton; 2002. p. 190-1.

90  Viscott D. *Emotionally Free: letting go of the past to live in the moment.* Chicago: NTC; 1992. p.9.

91  Viscott D. *Emotionally Free: letting go of the past to live in the moment.* Chicago: NTC; 1992. p.12.

92  Emery G. *A New Beginning: how you can change your life through cognitive therapy.* New York: Simon & Schuster; 1981. p. 54.

93  Emery G. *A New Beginning: how you can change your life through cognitive therapy.* New York: Simon & Schuster; 1981. p. 57-63.

94  Christian K. *Your Own Worst Enemy: breaking the habit of adult underachievement.* New York: Norton; 2002. p. 107-111.

95  Christian K. *Your Own Worst Enemy: breaking the habit of adult underachievement.* New York: Norton; 2002. p. 122-125.

96  Beck M. Receive with an open heart: giving and accepting gifts of real love. Beck [serial online] 2012 Aug. Available from: http://marthabeck.com/2012/08/receiving-open-heart/

97  Golabuk P. *Recovering from a Broken Heart.* New York: Harper and Row; 1989, p. 160-1.

98  Lyubomirsky S. *The How of Happiness: a scientific approach to getting the life you want.* [monograph online] New York: Penguin; 2008. p. 89.

99  Lyubomirsky S. *The How of Happiness: a scientific approach to getting the life you want.* [monograph online] New York: Penguin; 2008. p. 125-130.

100  Lyubomirsky S. *The How of Happiness: a scientific approach to getting the life you want.* [monograph online] New York: Penguin; 2008. p. 125-130.

101  Lyubomirsky S. *The How of Happiness: a scientific approach to getting the life you want.* [monograph online] New York: Penguin; 2008. p. 130- 133.

102  Lyubomirsky S. *The How of Happiness: a scientific approach to getting the life you want.* [monograph online] New York: Penguin; 2008. p. 92- 95.

103  The benefits of giving. Yahoo [serial online] 2013 Mar
Available from: http://voices.yahoo.com/the-benefits-giving-12043525.html?cat=48

104  Niven D. *The 100 Simple Secrets of Happy People.* [monograph online] New York: Harper Collins; 2009 Mar. p. 135.

[105] Niven D. *The 100 Simple Secrets of Happy People*. [monograph online] New York: Harper Collins; 2009 Mar. p. 140-1.

[106] Burns D. *The Feeling Good Handbook*. New York: Plume; 1999 May. p. 376-410.

[107] Volunteering. NHS [serial online] 2013 Aug. Available from: http://www.nhs.uk/livewell/volunteering/pages/volunteeringhome.aspx

[108] Why volunteer? NHS [serial online] 2013 Aug. Available from: http://www.nhs.uk/Livewell/volunteering/Pages/Whyvolunteer.aspx

[109] How to volunteer. NHS [serial online] 2013 Aug. Available from: http://www.nhs.uk/Livewell/volunteering/Pages/Howtovolunteer.aspx

[110] New years resolution statistics. Statisticbrain [serial online] 2014 Jan. Available from: http://www.statisticbrain.com/new-years-resolution-statistics/

[111] Robb A. Will you keep your New Year's resolutions? This data predicts your success. New Republic [serial online] 2013 Dec. Available from: http://www.newrepublic.com/node/116075/print

[112] Burns D. *The Feeling Good Handbook*. New York: Plume; 1999 May p. 92.

[113] Burns D. *The Feeling Good Handbook*. New York: Plume; 1999 May p. 96

[114] Burns D. *The Feeling Good Handbook*. New York: Plume; 1999 May p. 118-9

[115] Burns D. *The Feeling Good Handbook*. New York: Plume; 1999 May p. 172-3

[116] Burns D. *The Feeling Good Handbook*. New York: Plume; 1999 May p. 170-2

[117] Burns D. *The Feeling Good Handbook*. New York: Plume; 1999 May p. 183-206.

[118] Eat a Rainbow accessed in June 2018 http://www.nutritionaustralia.org/national/resource/eat-rainbow

[119] Stanger J. Why Whole Grains Should Be Part of Your Diet accessed in June 2018 at https://www.forksoverknives.com/why-whole-grains-should-be-part-of-your-diet/#gs.=CMjQPo

[120] Campbell, T. C., & Campbell, T. M. Revised and Expanded Edition. The China Study: The most comprehensive study of nutrition ever conducted and the startling implications for diet, weight loss and long-term health; 2016 p.60-88.

[121] Pulde, A. & Lederman. M. The Forks Over Knives Plan: How to Transition to the Life-Saving, Whole-Food, Plant-Based Diet ; 2017 p.10-15

Lightning Source UK Ltd.
Milton Keynes UK
UKHW020944270123
416051UK00009B/92

9 781982 280130